THE BIG BOOK OF PALEO COOKING

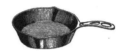

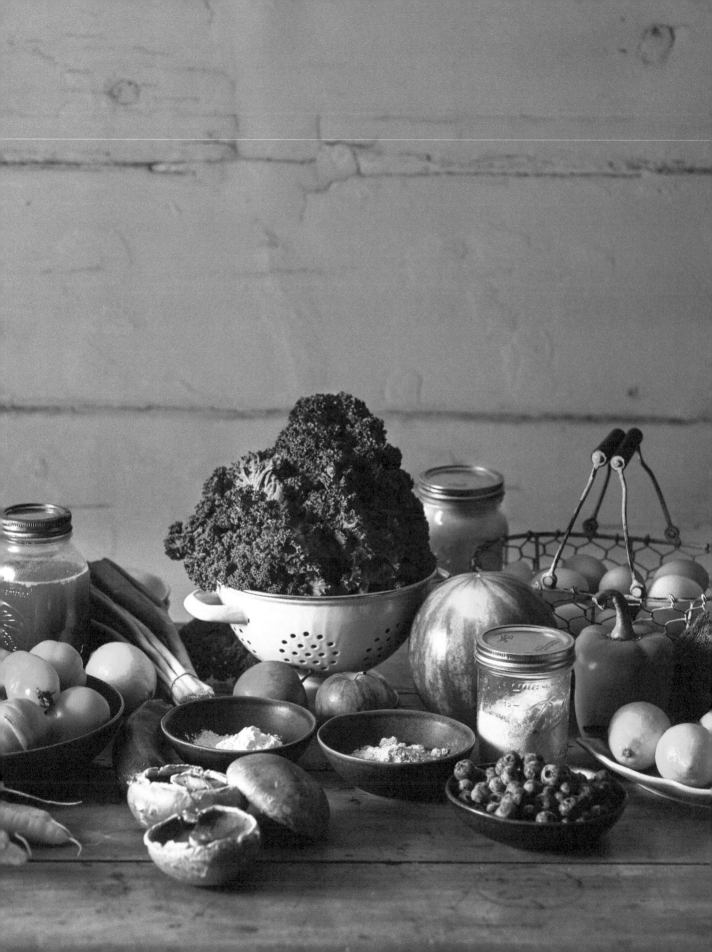

THE BIG BOOK OF
PALEO
COOKING

175 Recipes & 6 Weeks of Meal Plans

Angela Blanchard

Photography by Darren Muir

ROCKRIDGE
PRESS

Interior & Cover Designer: Francesca Pacchini
Art Producer: Maura Boland
Editor: Jesse Aylen
Production Editor: Nora Milman
Photography by © 2019 Darren Muir
Author Photo courtesy of ©JKL Images

Cover recipe: Pan-Seared Pork Chops (page 151)

ISBN: Print 978-1-64611-225-8 | eBook 978-1-64611-226-5
R0

This book is dedicated to Forest
and Hunter—I love you to the ocean and back.

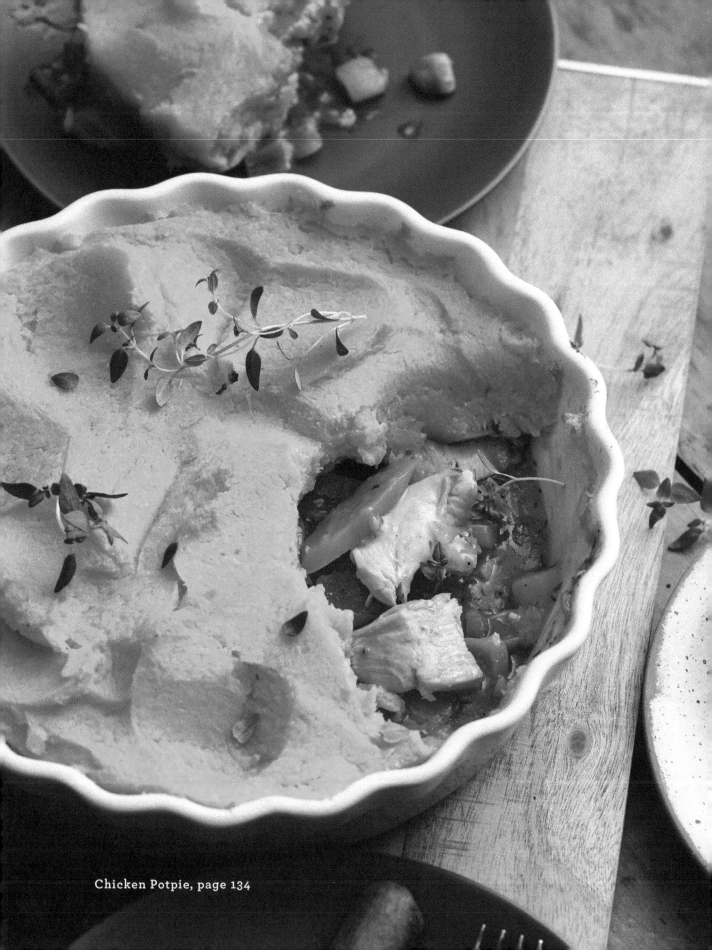

Chicken Potpie, page 134

CONTENTS

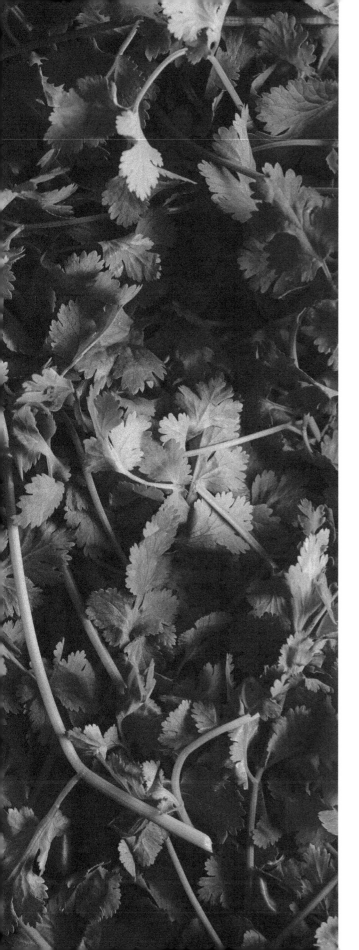

INTRODUCTION

For years, I struggled with infertility, extreme anxiety, bouts of depression, and being overweight. I chased diet fads, took weight-loss supplements, and participated in strenuous exercise programs. Yet I always ended up back where I started, only more tired, depressed, and hungrier than before.

After my second son was born, I finally realized my lifestyle habits were affecting not only me but my family as well. Like our genes, our habits get passed down from generation to generation. I started to break my family's chain of negative lifestyle practices by following the paleo diet.

I changed my diet one step at a time. I eliminated grains first, then dairy, legumes, refined sugars, and all things processed. Within the first week, I began to notice changes in my body and mental clarity: I was more energized, I was sleeping better, and for the first time in a long time, I felt happier.

As the weeks went on, I continued to progress. That first year I lost 54 pounds, and I have continued to maintain my weight through the paleo diet. I use the word *diet* very loosely throughout this book, as I see paleo more as a lifestyle than as a diet. Eating paleo is a sustainable way to live that promotes overall wellness and provides your mind and body with everything they need to be their very best.

Since I transitioned to paleo, it has been my mission to help others reap the benefits. Unfortunately, there are a lot of misconceptions about the paleo diet—everything from "It's too expensive to eat healthy" to "It's not sustainable for working families."

Eating paleo isn't expensive. When you ditch the prepackaged franken-foods, you save money and make room in your budget for healthier options. You'll likely notice a difference in your grocery bill once you replace those less healthy foods with fresh and whole paleo options.

When you transition away from a high-carb diet, your body depends less on glucose and more on its own stored fat for energy. As a result, you'll find yourself eating more nutrient-dense foods that keep you feeling fuller longer, but you'll be eating less frequently.

Eating paleo does not require more time to prepare meals. When it comes to eating healthier options, my favorite phrase is "keep it simple." Although there's a time and place for creative, healthy twists on traditional comfort foods, we don't need to eat like that every night. Mealtime can be as easy as having a chicken breast and two helpings of vegetables roasted or sautéed in coconut oil (or in my favorite—richly flavorful bacon drippings).

Once you are familiar with the ins and outs of paleo, you can easily plan your meals for the week ahead or follow the meal plans I've provided. By the end, you'll be an expert at planning, cooking, and eating everything paleo and have a firm grasp on how to make it work best for you.

The Big Book of Paleo Cooking takes you on an easy-to-follow journey that gives you everything you need to achieve your health and wellness goals. Whether you have an autoimmune disorder, want to lose weight, or want to eat healthier, there is a solution, recipe, and meal plan for every appetite. Together, we will get you there.

Happy eating!

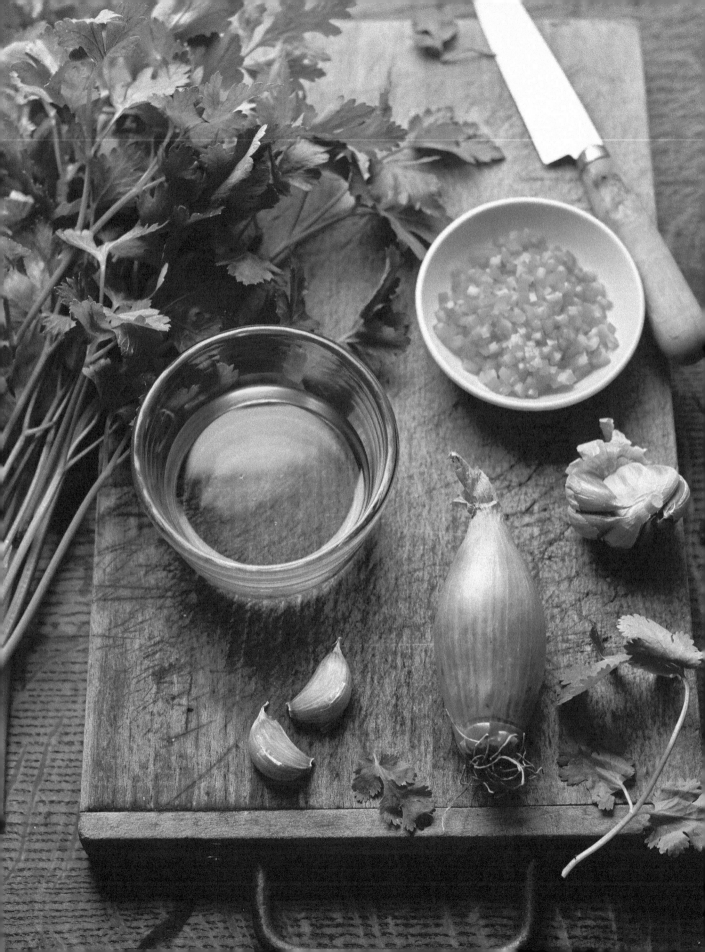

CHAPTER ONE

PLANNING YOUR PALEO SUCCESS

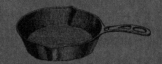

To be successful, you first need to understand the basics of the paleo diet. Knowing what you should and shouldn't eat will help you weed out those foods that have been plaguing you, whether you've realized it or not.

This section will help you better understand the paleo diet and prepare a well-stocked kitchen. Although there are some foods to avoid, there are plenty more to embrace. By the end of this chapter, you'll be able to turn any meal into a delicious experience using only fresh foods and your updated pantry.

THE PRINCIPLES OF PALEO

Paleo focuses on foods that give our bodies everything they need to thrive: meat, fowl, eggs, vegetables, fruits, nuts, seeds, and healthy fats. These foods provide the building blocks for success; nothing else is needed.

WHOLE FOODS: THE PALEO ESSENTIAL

The paleo diet focuses on whole, unprocessed foods as the foundation of every meal while eliminating grains, dairy, refined sugars, and legumes. Although some foods are more objectionable than others, it is crucial to follow the paleo diet in full. When you do, you're likely to see results, such as weight loss, clearer skin, and improved immune and gut health, much sooner. Quality and organic proteins, healthy fats, and organic vegetables and fruits should be the cornerstones of every meal, with a handful of nuts and seeds on occasion.

As healthier options are making their way into our supermarkets, finding minimally processed pantry staples is becoming easier. I encourage you to think of your paleo diet as adventurous. Start by replacing your baking flours with almond or coconut flour, then substitute dairy milks with full-fat coconut milk. Swap out refined sugars for natural sugars, such as raw honey or pure maple syrup, and get creative and indulgent by crafting special paleo desserts. Making these simple swaps will allow you to embrace change while incorporating exciting flavors and satisfaction into every meal.

WAVE GOODBYE TO WHEAT AND DAIRY

For some, consuming wheat and dairy can be problematic, from aggravating inflammation and compromised gut health to potentially causing digestive issues and creating weight-loss barriers.

Several dairy products such as yogurt, ice cream, butter, and cream contain refined sugars, chemical sweeteners, additives, and hormones. Instead of exposing yourself to these objectionable ingredients, avoid all dairy or purchase full-fat, minimally processed dairy products (cream, butter, cheese) if you do not have adverse effects. Some simple dairy replacements are coconut or tree nut–based milk, cheese, and butter products or ghee.

Grains are very addictive. Surprise! Did you notice when you transitioned from a grain-based diet to a paleo one that you faced some unpleasant side effects during the first week or two? Unfortunately, the fatigue, nausea, headaches, and withdrawal-like symptoms are all the result of a grain-based diet. Thankfully, these feelings last only a short time before you experience an overall improvement in digestion and inflammatory balance.

When it comes to grain-based products, find paleo-friendly companies for prepackaged or premade paleo versions. See the Resources for some of my favorite suggestions! Otherwise, replace your baking flour with almond, coconut, cassava, tigernut, or arrowroot flour to make one of the temptingly sweet creations found in these pages.

OIL OPTIONS

Not all fats are created equal. Despite conventional wisdom, saturated and monosaturated fats are excellent paleo-friendly sources of healthy caloric energy, and you can use saturated and monosaturated fats to cook and prepare paleo meals.

Saturated fats are found in animal-based foods, such as meat and eggs, as well as in coconut and palm oil. These fats are temperature stable. If you are frying or baking at high temperatures, use saturated fat as a flavor-boosting, paleo-friendly alternative to canola or vegetable oil.

Monosaturated fats, such as nut oil and olive oil, are paleo-friendly, but they should not be exposed to extreme heat. Other monosaturated fats, such as avocado and extra-virgin olive oil, make excellent bases for condiments and dressings.

Avoid fake butter spreads and canola, soy, corn, safflower, and sunflower oils. These oils, also known as polyunsaturated fats, have been researched as potential culprits for a range of chronic health issues. Polyunsaturated fats contain more fluid, which allows them to remain in liquid form regardless if they're stored in the pantry or refrigerator. These fats are not temperature stable and may cause widespread inflammation, even if you're exposed to only small amounts.

LOVE IT OR LOSE IT

Utilize the following lists for a better understanding of which foods to embrace and which ones to avoid. It's best to purchase quality proteins and healthy fats and focus on organic or local products when available. Shop the perimeter of the store and avoid walking down the aisles. My general rule is if you can hunt or grow it, you can eat it. The list of foods to love is just a general guideline; there are plenty of other options!

FOODS TO LOVE

Dig into these paleo-friendly foods to keep yourself energized and full every day.

Beverages: water, herbal teas, coffee, nut-based milk, and homemade smoothies

Carbohydrates: nut- and tuber-based flours and butters from coconuts, almonds, tapioca, cassava, arrowroot, and tigernuts

Fats and oils: lard, tallow, ghee, coconut oil, palm oil/shortening, avocado oil, macadamia oil, and extra-virgin olive oil

Fruits: blackberries, blueberries, bananas, strawberries, apples, apricots, cherries, figs, kiwi, limes, oranges, peaches, pineapple, watermelon, grapefruit, coconut, mango, and grapes

Protein: chicken, duck, fowl, eggs, turkey, beef, pork, lamb, bison, elk, goat, pheasant, rabbit, venison, freshwater fish, shellfish, and seafood

Sugars: raw and unfiltered honey, pure grade A maple syrup, coconut sugar, monk fruit, and stevia

Vegetables: kale, spinach, lettuce, collard greens, asparagus, avocados, beets, peppers, broccoli, Brussels sprouts, cabbage, carrots, tomatoes, celery, and winter and summer squashes

FOODS TO LOSE

Avoid these foods to ensure your paleo success.

Grain-based carbohydrates: all grains (wheat, rye, corn, barley, oats, etc.), legumes (lentils, peanuts, beans, chick-peas, and soy), and processed foods (breakfast cereals, cake mixes, microwave meals, pasta, snacks, crackers, donuts, etc.)

Nonorganic fruits: canned fruits that are preserved with chemicals and sugar, fruits that are conventionally grown (using fertilizers and pesticides) and difficult to wash or peel

Nonorganic vegetables: canned vegetables preserved with chemicals and sugar, vegetables that are conventionally grown (using fertilizers and pesticides) and difficult to wash or peel

Polyunsaturated fats/oils: fake butter spreads and canola, soy, corn, safflower, and sunflower oils

Processed protein: designer meats such as hot dogs, deli meats, breakfast sausages, and those from concentrated animal-feeding operations

Refined sugars: table sugar, brown sugar, corn syrup, processed syrups and honey, agave, and hidden sugars in sauces, dressings, coffees, soups, and smoothies

Sweetened beverages: soda, sports drinks, sweetened nut-based and yogurt-based milk and smoothies, flavored waters, juices from concentrate, and energy drinks

Considering Cholesterol on Paleo

Modern guidelines regarding cholesterol are solely based on prepackaged, modified, and chemical-tinged foods from the standard American diet. If you're currently experiencing elevated or increased cholesterol levels and are concerned about adopting the paleo diet, I encourage you to check with your healthcare professional about monitoring your cholesterol while you're following the paleo diet.

YOUR PALEO PANTRY

A smartly stocked pantry is your kitchen's best asset since it ensures you have everything you need to make paleo meals. You don't need to throw away everything at once. Start by swapping out flours or adding natural sugars and work your way up to a fully functional paleo pantry. Here are some items you'll need to prepare the meals in this book:

Almond butter

Apple cider vinegar

Arrowroot flour

Avocado oil

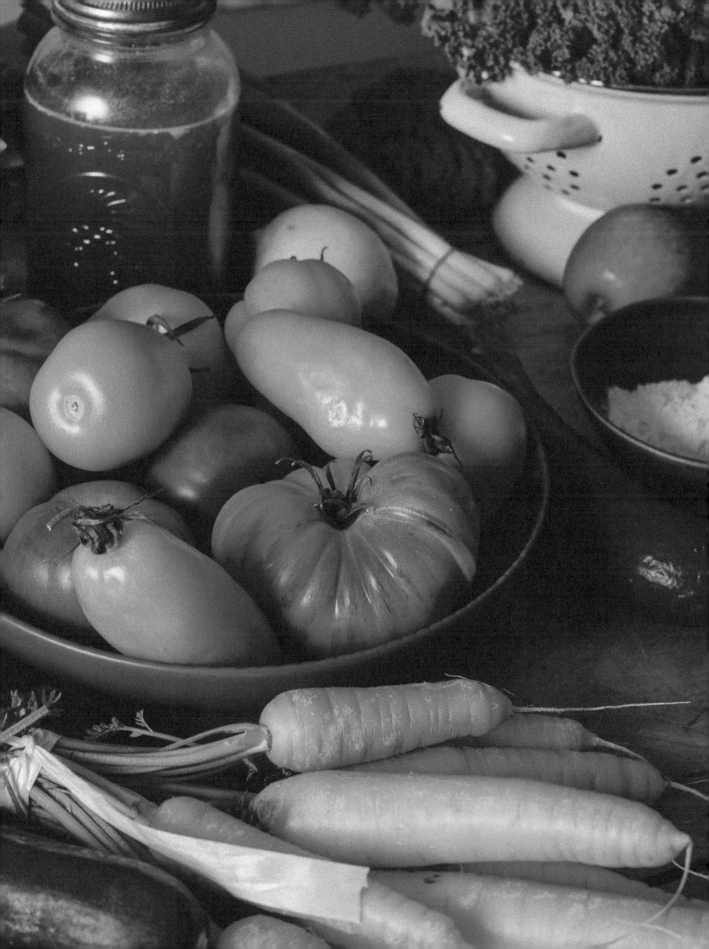

Blanched almond flour

Cacao powder

Canned coconut milk

Canned tomatoes (paste, sauce, diced)

Coconut aminos

Coconut flour

Coconut oil

Coconut sugar

Extra-virgin olive oil

Pecans

Pure maple syrup

Raw honey

Shredded coconut

Spices (garlic powder, onion powder, chili powder, oregano, cinnamon, paprika, salt, pepper, etc.)

Vanilla extract

Walnuts

These are my top pantry staples. You can use them in just about any recipe, and most paleo recipes call for some of these ingredients. All of them should be available at your local supermarket. Double-check the ingredient lists, though, to make sure there are no hidden sugars or unnecessary ingredients.

Many of the recipes in this book have tips for ingredient replacements to ensure there are options for everyone, whether you follow a strict autoimmune protocol (AIP) diet or have allergies to one or more of the ingredients.

Paleo After-Hours

Unless you are following the paleo diet for strictly medical reasons, indulging in an occasional adult beverage (or two) is okay. Despite the misconception, drinking an occasional—emphasis on *occasional*—alcoholic beverage does not have to undermine your paleo-driven health goals.

From a paleo perspective, your first choice for an alcoholic beverage should always be a quality red or white wine because it's not grain-based and provides some healthy antioxidants. Most spirits, such as whiskey, tequila, and vodka, have zero carbohydrates. Although the distillation process removes most of the gluten, it's still present in trace amounts, which can be a concern for paleo imbibers. Skip mixed drinks made with spirits and opt for straight spirits served over ice instead.

Lastly, if you must drink beer, opt for lighter options as they are lower in carbohydrates, and avoid regular, stout, and microbrews. Since alcohol has no nutritional value and disrupts digestion and nutrient absorption, it can hinder weight-loss efforts and personal health goals. Practice responsible moderation and avoid excess.

KEEP IT SWEET THE PALEO WAY

Although an occasional sweet treat is okay, we shouldn't eat desserts (paleo or otherwise) daily.

Because of their nutritional value, natural sweeteners are healthier than heavily refined table sugar and brown sugar, but all sugar is broken down the same regardless of its origin. The most easily sourced, paleo-friendly natural sweeteners are pure maple syrup, raw honey, and coconut sugar. Some paleo recipes call for other natural sweeteners such as stevia or erythritol, but I prioritize the most common and natural options throughout these recipes.

When swapping out refined sugars for paleo-approved sweeteners, use half of what the recipes require. For example, if a recipe calls for 1 cup of table sugar, use ½ cup of honey, maple syrup, or coconut sugar.

When you transition to the paleo diet, you'll notice that your taste buds become more sensitive to sugar, so I highly suggest playing around with recipes until you get the sweetness right.

KEEP IT COOL THE PALEO WAY

Like a well-stocked pantry, a full refrigerator ensures you can make a paleo meal at any moment and allows you to prep meals so you can cook effortlessly and efficiently.

Fresh vegetables are a must in every kitchen. To save time, I always wash, dry, cut, and store my produce in advance. Ready-to-eat vegetables ensure less prep work and provide a healthy grab-and-go snack.

Pasture-raised eggs, from your local farm or grocery store, have a rich taste and color and are always good to have on hand. If you cannot find pasture-raised eggs, the next best option is free-range or organic.

Uncured sugar-free bacon should be a staple in every household. Bacon has a high protein-to-fat ratio, making it one of the best animal fats. After cooking with bacon, strain and save the bacon grease for sautéing and roasting other dishes to bring even more flavor to your complementary sides.

Other refrigerator essentials include sauerkraut, hot sauce, and fish sauce. These ingredients let you add the right punch of sour, hot, and bold umami flavors to your dishes.

Paleo Comforts

In the early days of beginning your paleo diet, you may miss high-carbohydrate foods. Use these examples to find paleo-friendly alternatives to satisfy your cravings.

BREAD is a staple in many households, but there are so many options for bread substitutes. Get creative! Wrap sandwich contents in lettuce. Make buns out of sweet potatoes, mushroom caps, and eggs, or make my favorite homemade Almond Flour Bread (page 30) or AIP/Allergen-Free Tortillas (page 36).

POTATOES, most traditionally white and yellow ones, are found on dinner plates around the globe, but they're not so paleo friendly. When swapping out white and yellow potatoes, opt for sweet potatoes, which have a lower glycemic index and provide more nutrition.

RICE AND NOODLES make their way into many dishes. Luckily, there are a few companies that provide paleo options. If you are looking for a low-carbohydrate homemade option, Grated Cauliflower Rice (page 37) and Zucchini Noodles (Zoodles, page 32) make great alternatives.

LEGUMES (peanuts, beans, lentils, peas, and soy) should be avoided on the paleo diet. Although there is no direct substitute for legumes, consider adding extra meat or sweet potatoes to a recipe. Swap out your peanut butter for almond or cashew butter, and use coconut aminos as a soy sauce replacement.

BAKED GOODS have become a comfort food rather than a special treat at birthday parties. Ditch the store-bought baked goods, and make a delicious paleo alternative to your favorite dessert from the Sweets chapter (page 211).

ESSENTIAL EQUIPMENT

You'll only need a few kitchen tools to execute many of my recipes. You probably already have most of these items, and if you don't, they are relatively inexpensive.

Cast iron skillet: A cast iron skillet is hardy and versatile. You can use it on the grill or stove, in the oven, or even over the fire without ruining it.

Food processor: I use my food processor for many things, from puréeing to mixing. A standard eight-cup food processor will keep prep to a minimum.

Slow cooker: I'm all about cooking efficiently and effortlessly, and the slow cooker is my favorite kitchen item. Prep your meal the night before, turn it on the following morning, and have dinner ready as soon as you walk in the door.

NICE-TO-HAVE EQUIPMENT

Although it's possible to use more commonly available tools, these are helpful to have on hand if your budget and space allow.

Dutch oven: Perfect for a range of roasting and baking needs, the Dutch oven is a workhorse and kitchen stalwart.

Grill: When taking on the range of delicious proteins included in these recipes, a grill makes perfect sense, should your budget and space allow for it.

Mandoline: A mandoline makes short work of slicing vegetables, making prep speedy and simple.

Spiralizer: For spiralizing veggies to replace those bowls full of pasta you used to enjoy, a spiralizer is just about indispensable.

ABOUT THE RECIPES

In this book, you will find a dish for every occasion. Each recipe has easy-to-read nutritional information, a list of easily sourced ingredients, and simple instructions. At the end of every recipe, you will find useful tips, such as how to prep in advance and what substitutions to choose for allergen-free and AIP-friendly options. In the next chapter, I will offer helpful meal plans that address weight loss, the autoimmune protocol, and allergen-free options. A meal plan is an excellent tool, especially for those transitioning to the paleo diet or dealing with weight issues, autoimmune disorders, or allergies.

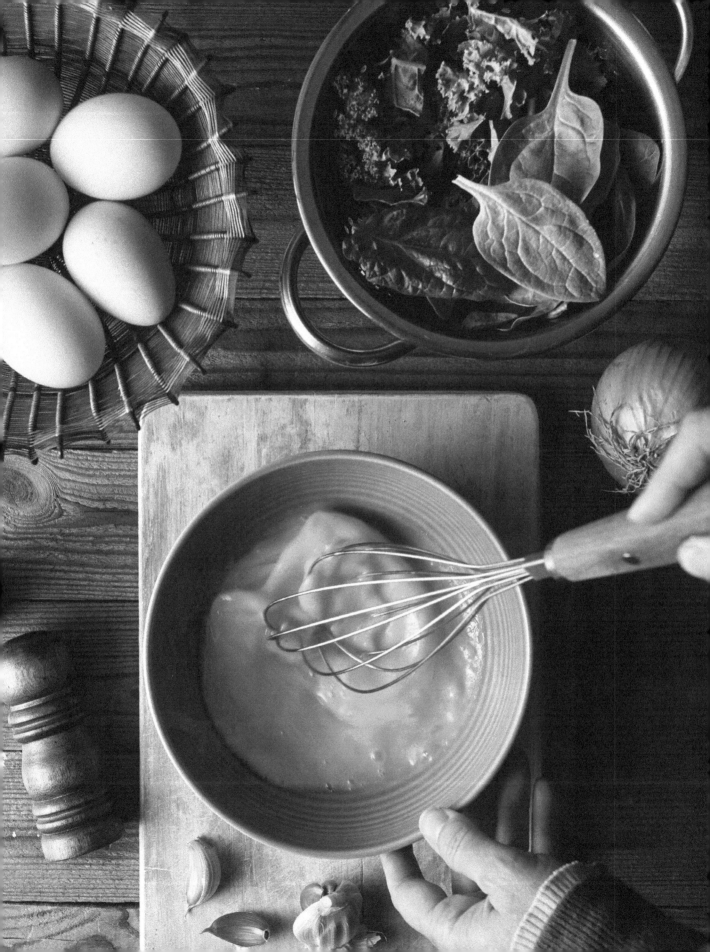

CHAPTER TWO

THE MEAL PLANS

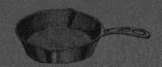

The paleo diet provides plenty of nutritional foods to choose from, so having a healthy balance in your macronutrients (protein, fats, and carbs) is accessible and sustainable. When you eat the paleo way to manage health-related issues, balance and customization are even more critical. These consecutive 14-day meal plans will provide guidance as you confront different challenges in weight loss, food allergies, and autoimmunity. As with any way of eating, your individual choice is vital. Use these meal plans in their entirety or as an inspirational structure within your personal routine. The morning boost and evening snack are optional, but they can be great options for individuals who are transitioning to the diet. Often, the first two weeks are the hardest as the gut heals itself, and these plans can help you navigate any feelings of deprivation.

WEIGHT LOSS

Packed with caloric energy and macronutrients, these recipes will have you feeling satisfied without starving yourself. Not everyone requires the same macronutrient ratios, but a great place to start is to consume 65 percent fat, 15 percent protein, and 20 percent carbohydrates. If you're fighting hunger pangs or decreased energy, try raising your protein and fiber intake and increasing your water consumption.

WEEK 1

	MONDAY	TUESDAY	WEDNESDAY
MORNING BOOST	Green tea	Bulletproof Coffee (page 72)	Warm water
MEAL #1	Denver-Style Egg Bake (page 42) and ½ avocado	Leftover Denver-Style Egg Bake (page 42) and ¼ cup berries	Mushroom and Chive Omelet (page 47) and Fresh Herbed Breakfast Sausages (page 59)
MEAL #2	Bang-Bang Shrimp Tacos (page 112)	Slow-Cooker Beef Roast with Gravy (page 178)	Pork Fried "Rice" (page 153)
EVENING ENDING	Carrots, celery, and 3 tablespoons almond butter	2 ounces dark chocolate	¼ cup almonds
DRINK	Water	Almond milk	Seltzer or club soda

Simple Snacks

If you missed a meal or need a midafternoon pick-me-up, try one of these nutrient-dense snacks that are also weight loss friendly:

Boiled eggs

Fresh fruit

Handful of tree nuts (almonds, cashews, pecans, walnuts)

Nitrate-Free Beef Jerky (page 203)

Nature's Trail Mix (page 204)

Sliced vegetables

THURSDAY	FRIDAY	SATURDAY	SUNDAY
Kombucha (page 83)	Green Machine Smoothie (page 76)	Green tea	Bulletproof Coffee (page 72)
Avocado Egg Tankers (page 51) and ¼ cup berries	Bacon and Egg Breakfast Burrito (page 53) and ½ avocado	Kitchen Sink Scrambler (page 46) and ¼ cup berries	Sausage and Spinach Egg Muffins (page 49)
Chimichurri Baked Chicken Breast (page 131) and Hasselback Sweet Potatoes (page 195)	Southwest Chili (page 101)	Sweet Citrus Pan-Seared Scallops (page 105) and Strawberry-Walnut Summer Salad (page 90)	Two-Meats Loaf (page 170) and Mashed Parsnips and Chives (page 198)
Bell peppers, cucumbers, and 3 tablespoons Roasted Cauliflower and Red Pepper Hummus (page 208)	¼ cup cashews	½ avocado and 1 tablespoon Creamy Ranch Dressing (page 236)	2 pieces Chocolate, Almond, and Sea Salt Fudge (page 223)
Herbal tea	Bone Broth (page 27 or 28)	Water	Almond milk

WEEK 2

	MONDAY	TUESDAY	WEDNESDAY
MORNING BOOST	Warm water	Kombucha (page 83)	Green Machine Smoothie (page 76)
MEAL #1	Turkey and Avocado Egg Wrap (page 43) and ¼ cup berries	Crustless Italian Breakfast Quiche (page 44) and ½ avocado	Leftover Crustless Italian Breakfast Quiche (page 44) and ¼ cup berries
MEAL #2	Shrimp Scampi (page 109)	Grilled Skirt Steak Fajitas (page 186)	Dry-Rubbed Ribs (page 145) and Roasted Honey-Mustard Sweet Potato Salad (page 209)
EVENING ENDING	¼ cup olives	¼ cup Nature's Trail Mix (page 204)	Carrots, celery, and 3 tablespoons almond butter
DRINK	Herbal tea	Bone Broth (page 27 or 28)	Water

THURSDAY	FRIDAY	SATURDAY	SUNDAY
Green tea	Bulletproof Coffee (page 72)	Warm water	Kombucha (page 83)
Sunrise Eggs Over Ham (page 48) and ½ avocado	Garlic, Spinach, and Kale Omelet (page 41) and Fresh Herbed Breakfast Sausages (page 59)	Spinach and Egg Stuffed Peppers (page 50) and ½ avocado	Good Morning Nachos (page 52)
Crispy Baked Chicken Thighs (page 127) and Maple Acorn Squash (page 202)	Italian Meatballs (page 191) and Garden-Fresh Spaghetti Sauce (page 240)	Lobster Alfredo (page 118)	Grilled Buffalo Chicken Salad (page 93) and Creamy Ranch Dressing (page 236)
¼ cup almonds	½ avocado and 1 tablespoon Creamy Ranch Dressing (page 236)	¼ cup cashews	Cinnamon Roll Mug Cake (page 216)
Almond milk	Seltzer or club soda	Herbal tea	Bone Broth (page 27 or 28)

AUTOIMMUNE AWARE

One plan can't address all autoimmune conditions. That said, this meal plan follows a very strict autoimmune protocol with a focus on anti-inflammatory foods. You will not find eggs, nuts, seeds, chocolate, coffee, nightshades, or any autoimmune offender in this AIP meal plan. It relies heavily on bone broths and recipes that utilize slow-cooked proteins and stews to minimize gastrointestinal flare-ups. The autoimmune protocol eliminates inflammatory foods to reset your immune system and heal your gut. After a few weeks, you can slowly start reintegrating foods into your diet to see if there is any adverse reaction. If you notice any side effects, take that food back out and continue to avoid it. Some individuals will adopt a strict AIP diet for life, while others can incorporate some foods back into their meals.

WEEK 1

	MONDAY	TUESDAY	WEDNESDAY
MORNING BOOST	Kombucha (page 83)	Bone Broth (page 27 or 28)	Warm water
MEAL #1	Cassava Waffles (page 66) and bacon	Apple-Cinnamon Porridge (page 64) and Fresh Herbed Breakfast Sausages (page 59)	Blueberry Pancakes (page 57) and bacon
MEAL #2	Classic Chicken Soup (page 100)	Baked Chimichurri Halibut (served with lemon wedge instead of chimichurri, page 108) and Bacon-Roasted Brussels Sprouts (page 196)	Zesty Italian Chicken and "Rice" Casserole (page 123)
EVENING ENDING	¼ cup berries	½ avocado	3 bacon slices
DRINK	Bone Broth (page 27 or 28)	Coconut milk	Herbal tea

Simple Snacks

If you missed a meal or need a midafternoon pick-me-up, try one of these AIP-friendly and nutrient-dense snacks:

AIP Granola Bars (page 62)
Avocados
Berries

Canned salmon or tuna
Dried fruit
Tigernuts

THURSDAY	FRIDAY	SATURDAY	SUNDAY
Coconut and Avocado Smoothie (page 75)	Green tea	Kombucha (page 83)	Bone Broth (page 27 or 28)
Sweet Potato Hash Browns (page 58) and Fresh Herbed Breakfast Sausages (page 59)	Coconut and Avocado Smoothie (page 75)	AIP Granola Bars (page 62) and ¼ cup berries	Turkey, Squash, and Apple Hash (page 140)
Slow-Cooked Beef Brisket (page 185)	Pan-Seared Pork Chops (page 151) and Maple Acorn Squash (page 202)	Creamy Cauliflower Soup (page 98)	Whole Herb-Roasted Turkey (page 125) and Hasselback Sweet Potatoes (page 195)
3 ounces tuna	AIP Granola Bars (page 62)	¼ cup olives	Mint Chip Ice Cream (page 220)
Water	Bone Broth (page 27 or 28)	Coconut water	Herbal tea

WEEK 2

	MONDAY	TUESDAY	WEDNESDAY
MORNING BOOST	Coconut and Avocado Smoothie (page 75)	Green tea	Kombucha (page 83)
MEAL #1	Sunrise Breakfast Hash (page 63)	Sweet Potato Toast (page 60) topped with jam	Cassava Waffles (page 66) and Fresh Herbed Breakfast Sausages (page 59)
MEAL #2	Chicken Potpie (page 134)	Perfectly Marinated Salmon (page 107)	Roasted Root Vegetables and Bacon (page 144)
EVENING ENDING	3 bacon slices	½ banana	¼ cup olives
DRINK	Herbal tea	Water	Bone Broth (page 27 or 28)

THURSDAY	FRIDAY	SATURDAY	SUNDAY
Bone Broth (page 27 or 28)	Glass warm water	Coconut and Avocado Smoothie (page 75)	Green tea
Coconut and Avocado Smoothie (page 75)	Blueberry Pancakes (page 57) and bacon	Turkey, Squash, and Apple Hash (page 140)	Fresh Herbed Breakfast Sausages (page 59) and fruit bowl
Beef Stroganoff (page 176)	Bacon-and-Apple-Stuffed Pork Chops (page 148)	Whole Roasted Lemon and Rosemary Chicken (prepared with coconut oil, page 124)	Cuban Braised Pork Shoulder (page 156)
¼ cup berries	½ avocado	AIP Granola Bars (page 62)	Banana Cream Pie Parfait (page 61)
Coconut water	Kombucha (page 83)	Herbal tea	Water

ALLERGEN-FRIENDLY

The recipes in this meal plan are entirely free from the top eight allergens: milk, eggs, fish, shellfish, tree nuts, peanuts, wheat, and soy. Whether you have a severe allergy to any of these or experience minimal symptoms such as acne, rashes, hives, and inflammation, this plan offers relief.

WEEK 1

	MONDAY	TUESDAY	WEDNESDAY
MORNING BOOST	Warm water	Bone Broth (page 27 or 28)	Coconut and Avocado Smoothie (page 75)
MEAL #1	Turkey, Squash, and Apple Hash (page 140)	Cassava Waffles (page 66) and bacon	Apple-Cinnamon Porridge (page 64) and Fresh Herbed Breakfast Sausages (page 59)
MEAL #2	Baja Chicken Fajitas (page 141)	Game Day Chili (page 179)	Pork Carnitas (page 161)
EVENING ENDING	2 ounces dark chocolate	AIP Granola Bars (page 62)	¼ cup berries
DRINK	Herbal tea	Coconut milk	Water

Simple Snacks

If you missed a meal or need a midafternoon pick-me-up, try one of these allergy-friendly and nutrient-dense snacks:

Avocado

Bacon

Dark chocolate (75 percent or higher cacao content)

Fresh fruits and vegetables

Olives

Sweet potato chips

THURSDAY	FRIDAY	SATURDAY	SUNDAY
Kombucha (page 83)	Green tea	Warm water	Bone Broth (page 27 or 28)
Blueberry Pancakes (page 57) and Fresh Herbed Breakfast Sausages (page 59)	Sweet Potato Toast (page 60) topped with jam	Coconut and Avocado Smoothie (page 75)	AIP Granola Bars (page 62) and ¼ cup berries
Sweet and Spicy Chicken Skewers (page 130)	Beef and Broccoli Stir-Fry (page 181)	Garden-Fresh Tomato and Basil Soup (page 94)	Sweet and Spicy Pork Belly Bites (page 154)
¼ cup olives	3 bacon slices	½ avocado	Mint Chip Ice Cream (page 220)
Bone Broth (page 27 or 28)	Coconut water	Herbal tea	Water

WEEK 2

	MONDAY	TUESDAY	WEDNESDAY
MORNING BOOST	Coconut and Avocado Smoothie (page 75)	Kombucha (page 83)	Green tea
MEAL #1	Sunrise Breakfast Hash (page 63)	Coconut and Avocado Smoothie (page 75)	Cassava Waffles (page 66) and bacon
MEAL #2	Zesty Italian Chicken and 'Rice' Casserole (page 123)	Barbecue Chicken and Pineapple (page 128)	Sloppy Joes (page 171)
EVENING ENDING	¼ cup olives	½ avocado	3 slices bacon
DRINK	Bone Broth (page 27 or 28)	Coconut water	Herbal tea

THURSDAY	FRIDAY	SATURDAY	SUNDAY
Warm water	Bone Broth (page 27 or 28)	Coconut and Avocado Smoothie (page 75)	Kombucha (page 83)
Apple-Cinnamon Porridge (page 64) and Fresh Herbed Breakfast Sausages (page 59)	Blueberry Pancakes (page 57) and Fresh Herbed Breakfast Sausages (page 59)	AIP Granola Bars (page 62) and ¼ cup berries	Sweet Potato Hash Browns (page 58) and Fresh Herbed Breakfast Sausages (page 59)
Korean Pork Chops (page 155) and Grated Cauliflower Rice (page 37)	Spicy Beef and Sweet Potatoes (page 187)	Roasted Portobello Mushroom Burgers (page 188)	Southwest Chili (page 101)
2 ounces dark chocolate	¼ cup berries	AIP Granola Bars (page 62)	Banana Cream Pie Parfait (page 61)
Water	Coconut milk	Bone Broth (page 27 or 28)	Coconut water

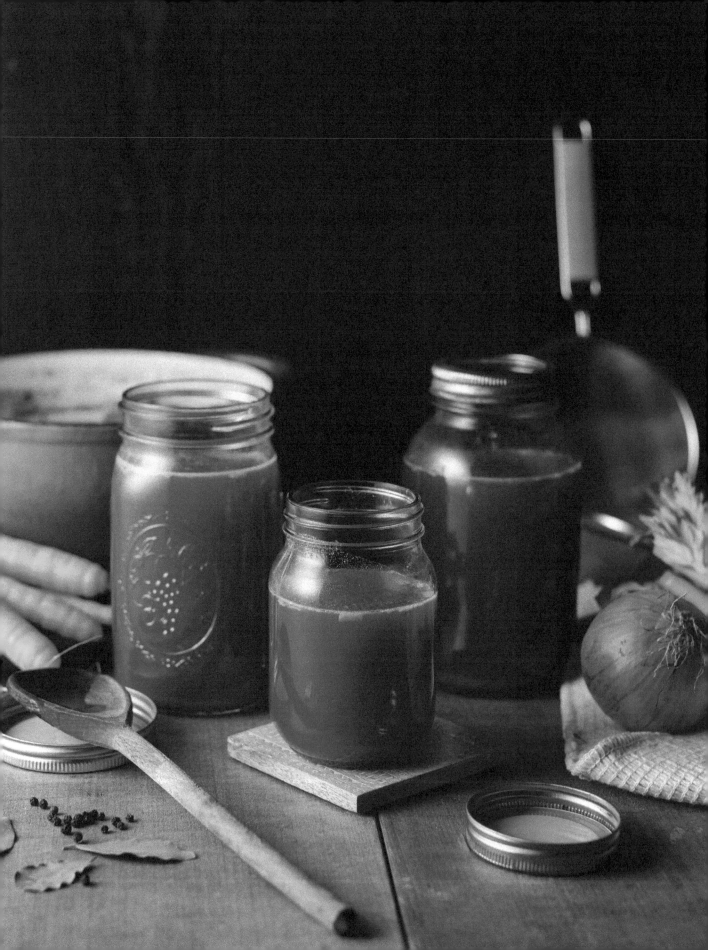

CHAPTER THREE

BASIC BROTHS AND CARB REPLACEMENTS

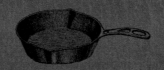

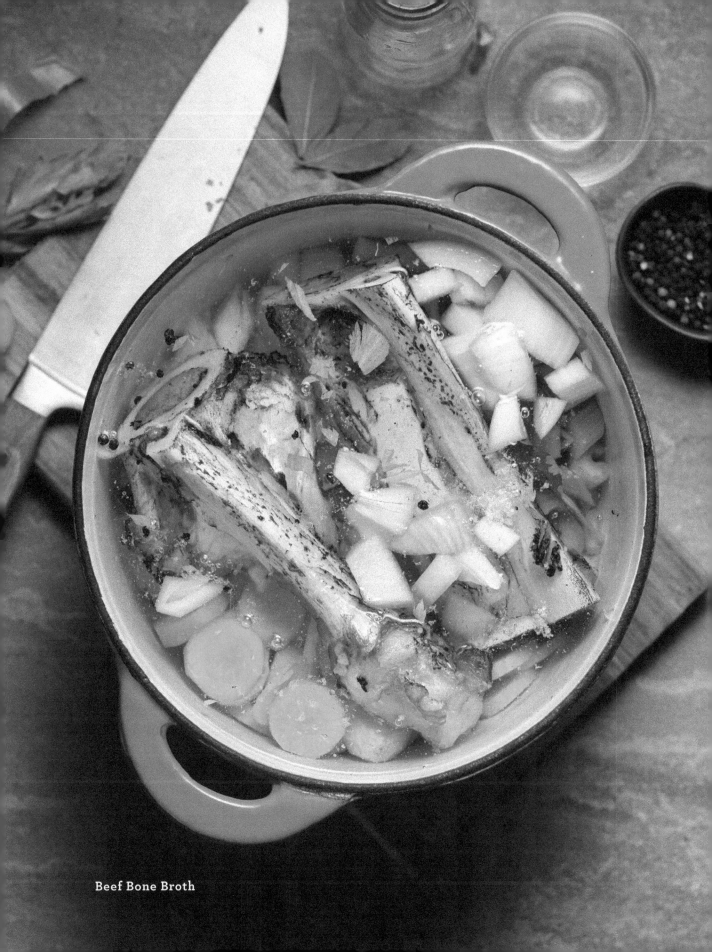

Beef Bone Broth

BEEF BONE BROTH

AIP-FRIENDLY, ALLERGEN-FREE, EASY, EGG-FREE, NUT-FREE

MAKES 6 TO 8 CUPS | PREP TIME: **15 MINUTES** | COOK TIME: **12 TO 24 HOURS, PLUS 1 HOUR TO COOL**

With every sip of this lush broth, you'll relish the vegetal sweetness and the earthiness of the beef bones with just enough spice to satisfy.

---

3 to 4 pounds mixed beef knuckles, joints, feet, and marrow bones

2 medium celery stalks, chopped

2 medium carrots, chopped

1 medium white onion, chopped

2 garlic cloves, peeled

1 bay leaf

1 teaspoon sea salt

1 teaspoon whole peppercorns

2 tablespoons apple cider vinegar

10 to 12 cups water

1. Preheat the oven to 400°F.

2. Place the beef bones in a single layer on a roasting pan or baking sheet and roast for 60 minutes, flipping the bones halfway through.

3. Put the celery, carrots, onion, garlic, bay leaf, salt, and peppercorns into a 6-quart or larger slow cooker.

4. Add the roasted bones, apple cider vinegar, and enough of the water to cover.

5. Cover and cook on low for 12 to 24 hours or until the broth is aromatic and a rich mahogany color.

6. Allow the broth to cool for 1 hour.

7. Carefully remove the bones and vegetables with a slotted spoon and discard.

8. Secure a piece of cheesecloth over a large bowl and slowly strain the broth.

9. Transfer the bone broth to an airtight container and store in the refrigerator for up to 2 weeks.

Storage Tip: For longer storage, freeze the broth in ice cube trays. Once the cubes are frozen, remove and place them in an airtight freezer-safe container or bag. One cube is roughly 1 ounce, so 8 cubes are equivalent to 1 cup of broth.

PER SERVING (1 CUP) CALORIES: 65; TOTAL FAT: 4G; SATURATED FAT: 1G; PROTEIN: 6G; TOTAL CARBOHYDRATES: 1G; FIBER: 0G; CHOLESTEROL: 0MG; MACROS: FAT: 55%; PROTEIN: 37%; CARBS: 8%

CHICKEN BONE BROTH

AIP-FRIENDLY, ALLERGEN-FREE, EASY, EGG-FREE, NUT-FREE

MAKES 6 TO 8 CUPS | PREP TIME: **15 MINUTES** | COOK TIME: **12 TO 24 HOURS, PLUS 1 HOUR TO COOL**

This chicken bone broth makes an excellent base for soups, but its smooth flavor can also be enjoyed on its own.

2 medium celery
   stalks, chopped

2 medium carrots, chopped

1 large white
   onion, chopped

2 garlic cloves, peeled

1 bunch fresh parsley

1 bay leaf

1 teaspoon sea salt

1 teaspoon
   whole peppercorns

Bones from 1 whole chicken

2 tablespoons apple
   cider vinegar

10 to 12 cups water

1. Put the celery, carrots, onion, garlic, parsley, bay leaf, sea salt, and peppercorns into a 6-quart or larger slow cooker.

2. Top with the chicken bones, apple cider vinegar, and enough of the water to cover.

3. Cover and cook on low for 12 to 24 hours or until the broth is aromatic and golden brown.

4. Allow the broth to cool for 1 hour.

5. Carefully remove the bones and vegetables with a slotted spoon and discard.

6. Secure a piece of cheesecloth over a large bowl and slowly strain the broth.

7. Transfer the bone broth to an airtight container and store in the refrigerator for up to 2 weeks.

Ingredient Tip: When making this broth, it's normal for the fat to float to the surface once it's cooled. You can leave it in the broth for rich and full flavor or skim it off to use the broth later in Classic Chicken Soup (page 100).

PER SERVING (1 CUP) CALORIES: 41; TOTAL FAT: 1G; SATURATED FAT: 0G; PROTEIN: 8G; TOTAL CARBOHYDRATES: 0G; FIBER: 0G; CHOLESTEROL: 0MG; MACROS: FAT: 21%; PROTEIN: 78%; CARBS: 1%

HOMEMADE ALMOND FLOUR

5 INGREDIENTS OR FEWER, EASY, EGG-FREE, QUICK PREP, UNDER 30 MINUTES

MAKES 2 CUPS | PREP TIME: **5 MINUTES**

Many of this book's recipes call for blanched almond flour thanks to its taste, texture, and how easy it is to work with compared to other paleo flours.

1 pound blanched and peeled almonds

1. In a food processor, pulse the almonds 50 to 60 times in 1-second increments or until the almonds are ground. Scrape the sides down as needed every 10 to 15 seconds.

2. Put the flour in an airtight container and store in the pantry until needed.

> Variation Tip: Save money and blanch almonds at home by soaking them in water overnight. Gently pinch the skin off the almonds and allow them to dry before grinding into flour.

PER SERVING (¼ CUP) CALORIES: 263; TOTAL FAT: 23G; SATURATED FAT: 2G; PROTEIN: 10G; TOTAL CARBOHYDRATES: 9G; FIBER: 5G; CHOLESTEROL: 0MG; MACROS: FAT: 73%; PROTEIN: 13%; CARBS: 14%

ALMOND FLOUR BREAD

EASY, QUICK PREP

MAKES 1 LOAF | PREP TIME: 10 MINUTES | COOK TIME: **1 HOUR**

I promise you'll want to slice into this hearty and nutrient-dense loaf for your next sandwich!

---

1 cup blanched almond flour (page 29)

¼ cup arrowroot flour

¼ cup tapioca flour

1 teaspoon baking soda

¼ teaspoon sea salt

3 large eggs

2 tablespoons apple cider vinegar

2 tablespoons extra-virgin olive oil

⅓ cup water

1. Preheat the oven to 350°F. Line a loaf pan with parchment paper.

2. In a large bowl, combine the almond, arrowroot, and tapioca flours, baking soda, and salt.

3. In a small bowl, whisk together the eggs, apple cider vinegar, olive oil, and water. Add the wet ingredients to the dry ingredients and stir until combined.

4. Pour the bread mixture into the prepared loaf pan and bake for 1 hour or until the bread has reached a deep, even golden brown color.

5. Remove the bread from the oven and cool completely before cutting.

> **Storage Tip:** Store the bread in an airtight container for up to 3 days on the counter or in the refrigerator.

PER SERVING (⅛ LOAF) CALORIES: 121; TOTAL FAT: 9G; SATURATED FAT: 1G; PROTEIN: 4G; TOTAL CARBOHYDRATES: 6G; FIBER: 1G; CHOLESTEROL: 70MG; MACROS: FAT: 67%; PROTEIN: 13%; CARBS: 20%

NO-OATS OATMEAL

SERVES 1 | PREP TIME: 3 MINUTES | COOK TIME: 2 MINUTES

Enjoy subtle hints of cinnamon mixed with the sweetness of a banana for a flavor-packed start to your morning, noon, or night.

½ medium banana

2 tablespoons blanched almond flour (page 29)

2 tablespoons unsweetened shredded coconut

1 tablespoon almond butter

⅓ cup full-fat coconut milk

¼ teaspoon ground cinnamon

1. In a small bowl, mash the banana using a fork until smooth.

2. Fold in the almond flour, coconut, almond butter, coconut milk, and cinnamon.

3. Microwave for 1 minute and 30 seconds or until the mixture starts to bubble.

4. Remove from the microwave and serve.

Variation Tip: For an allergen-free breakfast, try replacing the almond flour with 1 tablespoon of coconut flour and the almond butter with an equal amount of sunflower butter.

PER SERVING CALORIES: 487; TOTAL FAT: 39G; SATURATED FAT: 24G; PROTEIN: 8G; TOTAL CARBOHYDRATES: 26G; FIBER: 7G; CHOLESTEROL: 0MG; MACROS: FAT: 72%; PROTEIN: 7%; CARBS: 21%

ZUCCHINI NOODLES (ZOODLES)

5 INGREDIENTS OR FEWER, AIP-FRIENDLY, ALLERGEN-FREE, EASY, EGG-FREE, NUT-FREE, QUICK PREP, UNDER 30 MINUTES

SERVES 4 | PREP TIME: **5 MINUTES**

Zucchini noodles, also known as zoodles, are the perfect low-carbohydrate and gluten-free noodle alternative. Zoodles are an incredibly fresh substitute and a fun way to increase your vegetable intake.

1 large zucchini

1. Trim the ends off the zucchini.

2. Place the zucchini into a spiralizer and turn to create zucchini noodles.

3. Put the zoodles on a clean, dry towel and press to remove any excess moisture.

> Ingredient Tip: Zoodles can be eaten raw, sautéed, boiled, baked, or thrown into any dish!

PER SERVING CALORIES: 15; TOTAL FAT: 0G; SATURATED FAT: 0G; PROTEIN: 1G; TOTAL CARBOHYDRATES: 3G; FIBER: 1G; CHOLESTEROL: 0MG; MACROS: FAT: 1%; PROTEIN: 27%; CARBS: 72%

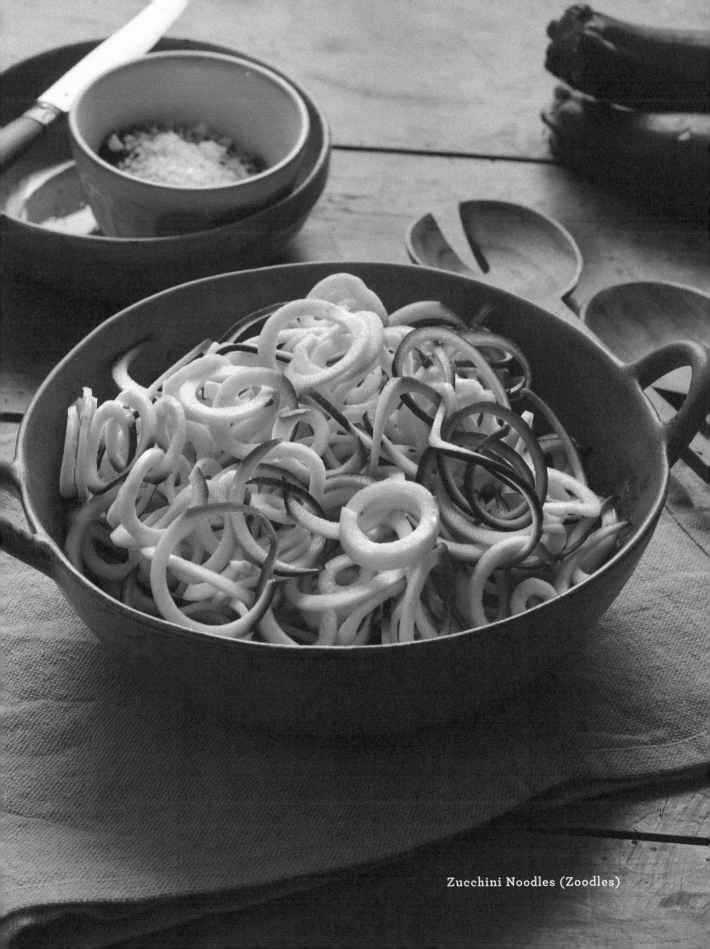

Zucchini Noodles (Zoodles)

MASHED SWEET POTATOES

5 INGREDIENTS OR FEWER, AIP-FRIENDLY, ALLERGEN-FREE, EASY, EGG-FREE, QUICK PREP

SERVES 4 | PREP TIME: **10 MINUTES** | COOK TIME: **20 MINUTES**

Swap out your traditional mashed potatoes for this simple, sweet, and low-glycemic alternative. This delicious recipe pairs well with any protein and makes a great holiday dinner side.

---

4 large sweet potatoes, peeled and cut into 1-inch chunks

½ cup full-fat coconut milk, more if needed

1 teaspoon sea salt

1 teaspoon freshly ground black pepper

1. Put the sweet potatoes into a medium stockpot with water to cover. Over medium-high heat, boil for 20 minutes or until the sweet potatoes are fork-tender.

2. Drain the potatoes and transfer them to a large bowl.

3. Add the coconut milk, salt, and pepper.

4. Using a potato masher or fork, mash for 1 minute or until smooth. (If the sweet potatoes are too thick, add coconut milk, a tablespoon at a time, until smooth and creamy.) Serve immediately.

Variation Tip: Coconut milk can be swapped out for almond milk.

PER SERVING CALORIES: 187; TOTAL FAT: 7G; SATURATED FAT: 6G; PROTEIN: 3G; TOTAL CARBOHYDRATES: 28G; FIBER: 5G; CHOLESTEROL: 0MG; MACROS: FAT: 34%; PROTEIN: 6%; CARBS: 60%

GRAIN-FREE PIZZA CRUST

EASY, EGG-FREE, QUICK PREP, UNDER 30 MINUTES

MAKES 1 (12-INCH) CRUST | PREP TIME: **10 MINUTES** | COOK TIME: **15 MINUTES**

This crust is the perfect foundation for any pizza. It has a texture similar to that of a traditional pizza crust with flavorful notes of oregano and garlic.

1 cup blanched almond flour (page 29)

¼ cup arrowroot flour

¼ cup flax meal

1 teaspoon garlic powder

1 teaspoon dried oregano

1 teaspoon cream of tartar

½ teaspoon sea salt

1 teaspoon baking soda

2 tablespoons apple cider vinegar

2 tablespoons extra-virgin olive oil

5 tablespoons warm water

1. Preheat the oven to 350°F.

2. In a large bowl, combine the almond flour, arrowroot flour, flax meal, garlic powder, oregano, cream of tartar, salt, and baking soda.

3. In a small bowl, whisk together the apple cider vinegar, olive oil, and water. Add the wet ingredients to the dry ingredients and stir until a soft ball of dough forms.

4. Allow the dough to rest for 5 minutes.

5. Place the dough between two large sheets of parchment paper and roll out with a rolling pin until the dough is ⅛ inch thick or as thin as desired without tearing the dough.

6. Slowly remove the top piece of parchment paper and transfer the dough with the bottom piece of parchment paper to a pizza pan or baking sheet.

7. Bake for 15 minutes or until golden brown and crisp. Allow to cool completely before topping.

Storage Tip: Cooked crust can be stored in the refrigerator for up to 5 days or in the freezer for up to 1 month. When ready to make your pizza, take the crust out and defrost it on the pizza pan or baking sheet you'll be cooking on.

PER SERVING (⅛ CRUST) CALORIES: 109; TOTAL FAT: 9G; SATURATED FAT: 1G; PROTEIN: 3G; TOTAL CARBOHYDRATES: 4G; FIBER: 2G; CHOLESTEROL: 0MG; MACROS: FAT: 74%; PROTEIN: 11%; CARBS: 15%

AIP/ALLERGEN-FREE TORTILLAS

5 INGREDIENTS OR FEWER, AIP-FRIENDLY, ALLERGEN-FREE, EASY, EGG-FREE, QUICK PREP, UNDER 30 MINUTES

MAKES 8 TORTILLAS | PREP TIME: 5 MINUTES | COOK TIME: **5 MINUTES**

You'll be able to enjoy this foolproof tortilla recipe regardless of your or your family's dietary restrictions.

1 cup cassava flour

¼ teaspoon sea salt

1 tablespoon coconut oil

8 to 10 tablespoons
    cool water

Coconut oil cooking spray

1. In a large bowl, combine the cassava flour and salt.

2. Add the coconut oil and knead the mixture for 1 minute or until crumbly. Add the water, 1 tablespoon at a time, while continuing to knead until a dough forms.

3. Divide the dough into 8 equal pieces and roll into 2-inch balls.

4. Place 1 ball between two sheets of parchment paper or plastic wrap and flatten using a tortilla press or rolling pin. Set aside, then repeat for each ball.

5. Grease a large skillet with cooking spray and heat over medium-high heat for 3 minutes or until the oil starts to shimmer.

6. Cook each tortilla for 2 minutes or until bubbles start to form. Flip and cook for an additional 2 minutes or until the edges start to fold up. Serve immediately.

> **Make-Ahead Tip:** Use these tortillas as the base for Beefy Taco Casserole (page 177) or Baja Chicken Fajitas (page 141).

PER SERVING CALORIES: 66; TOTAL FAT: 2G; SATURATED FAT: 2G; PROTEIN: 0G; TOTAL CARBOHYDRATES: 12G; FIBER: 2G; CHOLESTEROL: 0MG; MACROS: FAT: 27%; PROTEIN: 2%; CARBS: 71%

GRATED CAULIFLOWER RICE

5 INGREDIENTS OR FEWER, AIP-FRIENDLY, ALLERGEN-FREE, EASY, EGG-FREE, NUT-FREE, QUICK PREP, UNDER 30 MINUTES

SERVES 4 | PREP TIME: 5 MINUTES

Grated cauliflower is the perfect low-carbohydrate and low-calorie rice alternative. This fluffy reimagined "rice" can be used as a replacement in any dish that calls for rice.

1 large head cauliflower, cut into 1-inch florets

1. In a food processor, pulse the cauliflower 20 to 30 times or until it has a rice-like consistency.

2. Spread the grated cauliflower on a clean, dry towel and press to remove any excess moisture. Use immediately or store in the refrigerator for up to 3 days.

Variation Tip: Cauliflower can also be grated using a cheese grater.

PER SERVING CALORIES: 59; TOTAL FAT: 0G; SATURATED FAT: 0G; PROTEIN: 4G; TOTAL CARBOHYDRATES: 11G; FIBER: 5G; CHOLESTEROL: 0MG; MACROS: FAT: 1%; PROTEIN: 27%; CARBS: 72%

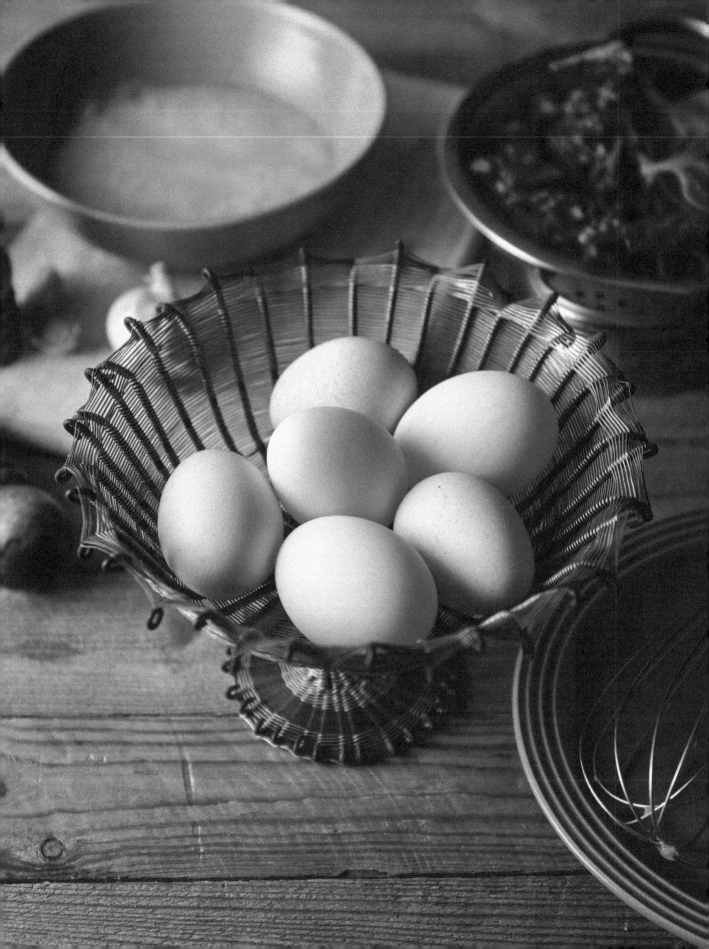

CHAPTER FOUR

UNBEATABLE EGGS

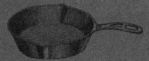

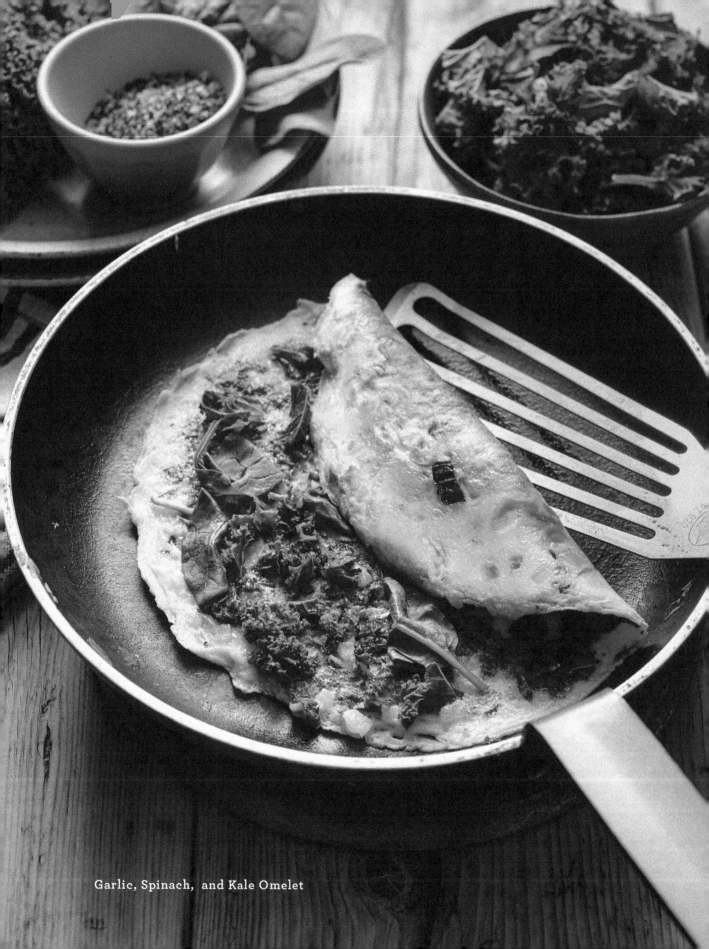

Garlic, Spinach, and Kale Omelet

GARLIC, SPINACH, AND KALE OMELET

EASY, NUT-FREE, QUICK PREP, UNDER 30 MINUTES

SERVES 1 | PREP TIME: 5 MINUTES | COOK TIME: 5 MINUTES

This punchy and flavorful omelet requires so little kitchen experience to whip up—it's sure to become a standby in your house.

---

1 tablespoon avocado oil

2 large eggs

1 garlic clove, minced

1 tablespoon finely chopped white onion

1 tablespoon chopped baby spinach

1 tablespoon chopped kale

Sea salt

Freshly ground black pepper

1. Heat the avocado oil in an 8-inch skillet over medium-high heat for 3 minutes or until the oil starts to shimmer.

2. In a small bowl, whisk the eggs.

3. Add the garlic and onion to the skillet and sauté for 1 to 2 minutes or until softened.

4. Add the spinach and kale and stir for 20 to 30 seconds or until partially wilted.

5. Add the whisked eggs and gently tilt the skillet back and forth until the eggs coat the pan evenly.

6. Season with salt and pepper.

7. Cook for 2 minutes or until the eggs are no longer visibly runny.

8. Carefully flip the eggs with a spatula without breaking them and cook for an additional 2 minutes or until firm.

> **Variation Tip:** Fresh garlic can be swapped out for ½ teaspoon of garlic powder.

PER SERVING CALORIES: 280; TOTAL FAT: 24G; SATURATED FAT: 5G; PROTEIN: 13G; TOTAL CARBOHYDRATES: 3G; FIBER: 0G; CHOLESTEROL: 372MG; MACROS: FAT: 77%; PROTEIN: 19%; CARBS: 4%

DENVER-STYLE EGG BAKE

EASY, QUICK PREP

SERVES 4 TO 6 | PREP TIME: 10 MINUTES | COOK TIME: **40 MINUTES**

Treat yourself to a Denver-style egg dish that's great for busy mornings or a large family brunch.

1 tablespoon avocado oil

½ medium white onion, finely chopped

½ red bell pepper, finely chopped

12 large eggs

⅓ cup almond milk

½ teaspoon sea salt

½ teaspoon freshly ground black pepper

1½ cups chopped nitrate- and sugar-free ham

¼ cup nutritional yeast

1. Preheat the oven to 400°F. Line a 9-by-13-inch baking dish with parchment paper.

2. Heat the avocado oil in a small skillet over medium-high heat for 3 minutes or until the oil starts to shimmer.

3. Sauté the onion and bell pepper for 3 minutes or until the vegetables are soft. Remove from the heat and set aside.

4. In a large bowl, whisk together the eggs, almond milk, salt, and pepper.

5. Arrange the sautéed onion and pepper and the ham in the prepared baking dish and pour in the egg mixture.

6. Sprinkle with nutritional yeast.

7. Bake for 30 to 35 minutes or until the middle of the egg bake is set and firm to the touch.

8. Remove the egg bake from the oven and cool before cutting and serving.

Ingredient Tip: Should you have it, use leftover Honey-Orange Glazed Ham (page 157) for this recipe.

PER SERVING CALORIES: 461; TOTAL FAT: 29G; SATURATED FAT: 11G; PROTEIN: 36G; TOTAL CARBOHYDRATES: 14G; FIBER: 6G; CHOLESTEROL: 587MG; MACROS: FAT: 57%; PROTEIN: 31%; CARBS: 12%

TURKEY AND AVOCADO EGG WRAP

EASY, NUT-FREE, QUICK PREP, UNDER 30 MINUTES

SERVES 1 | PREP TIME: 5 MINUTES | COOK TIME: 5 MINUTES

Ditch the traditional breakfast and start your day off right with this nutrient-dense and delicious turkey and avocado creation.

1 tablespoon avocado oil

2 large eggs

Sea salt

Freshly ground black pepper

1 slice nitrate- and sugar-free turkey

¼ medium avocado, sliced

1. Heat the avocado oil in an 8-inch skillet over medium-high heat for 3 minutes or until the oil starts to shimmer.

2. In a small bowl, whisk the eggs.

3. Pour the eggs into the skillet and gently tilt the skillet back and forth until the eggs coat the pan evenly.

4. Season with salt and pepper.

5. Cook the eggs for 2 minutes or until no longer visibly runny.

6. Carefully flip the eggs with a spatula without breaking them and cook for an additional 2 minutes or until firm.

7. Transfer to a plate, top with the turkey and avocado, and roll into a wrap.

> **Ingredient Tip:** If you have it on hand, use leftover Whole Herb-Roasted Turkey (page 125) for this recipe.

PER SERVING CALORIES: 387; TOTAL FAT: 31G; SATURATED FAT: 6G; PROTEIN: 20G; TOTAL CARBOHYDRATES: 7G; FIBER: 3G; CHOLESTEROL: 387MG; MACROS: FAT: 72%; PROTEIN: 21%; CARBS: 7%

CRUSTLESS ITALIAN BREAKFAST QUICHE

EASY, QUICK PREP

SERVES 4 TO 6 | PREP TIME: **10 MINUTES** | COOK TIME: **45 MINUTES, PLUS 5 MINUTES TO SET**

Enjoy hints of oregano, basil, and thyme with this light and flavorful low-carb quiche.

6 large eggs

1 cup full-fat coconut milk

1 tablespoon Zesty Italian Seasoning (page 232)

½ teaspoon sea salt

½ teaspoon freshly ground black pepper

¼ cup chopped broccoli florets

¼ cup finely chopped bell pepper

¼ cup chopped tomatoes

¼ cup chopped scallions, white and green parts

1. Preheat the oven to 350°F. Line a 9-inch pie dish with parchment paper.

2. In a medium bowl, whisk together the eggs, coconut milk, Italian seasoning, salt, and pepper.

3. Fold in the broccoli, bell pepper, tomatoes, and scallions.

4. Pour the mixture into the prepared pie dish and bake for 40 to 45 minutes or until the top is golden and the middle is firm to the touch. Let set for 5 minutes before cutting and serving.

> **Variation Tip:** Full-fat coconut milk can be swapped out for almond milk.

PER SERVING CALORIES: 275; TOTAL FAT: 23G; SATURATED FAT: 15G; PROTEIN: 11G; TOTAL CARBOHYDRATES: 6G; FIBER: 2G; CHOLESTEROL: 281MG; MACROS: FAT: 75%; PROTEIN: 16%; CARBS: 9%

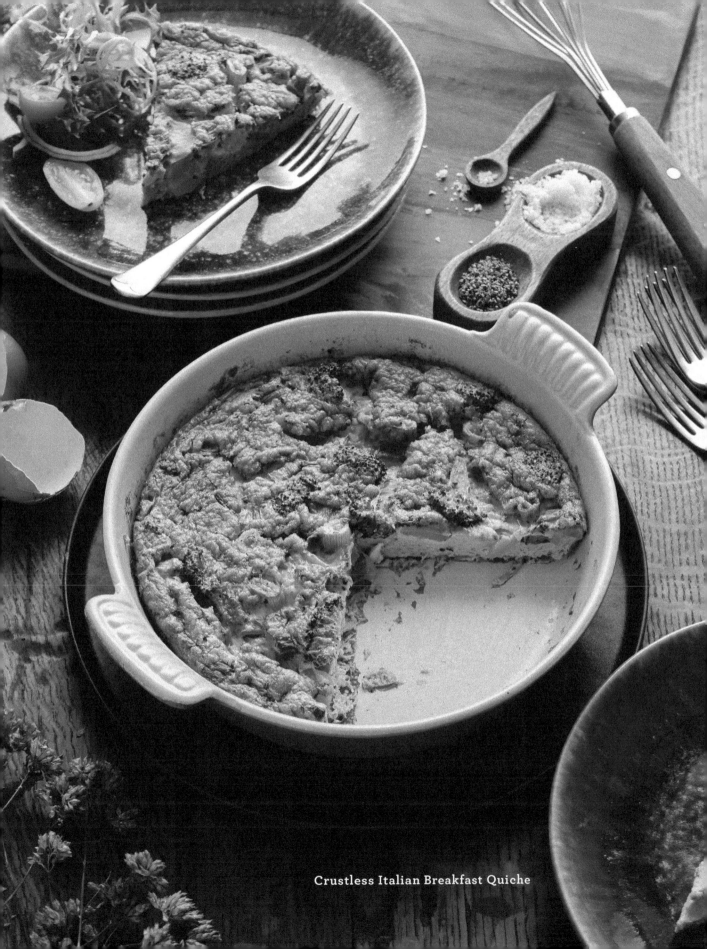

Crustless Italian Breakfast Quiche

KITCHEN SINK SCRAMBLER

EASY, NUT-FREE, QUICK PREP, UNDER 30 MINUTES

SERVES 1 | PREP TIME: 5 MINUTES | COOK TIME: 10 MINUTES

In my previous life as a health store line cook, this kitchen sink scrambler was one of my favorite dishes thanks to its well-balanced range of veggies.

---

2 large eggs

2 nitrate- and sugar-free bacon slices, chopped

1 tablespoon finely chopped white onion

1 tablespoon finely chopped mushrooms

1 tablespoon finely chopped bell pepper

1 tablespoon chopped baby spinach

Sea salt

Freshly ground black pepper

1. In a small bowl, whisk the eggs. Set aside.

2. Cook the bacon in an 8-inch skillet over medium-high heat for 3 minutes or until it starts to release its fat.

3. Add the onion, mushrooms, and bell pepper. Sauté for 3 minutes or until the bacon is brown and the vegetables are soft.

4. Add the spinach and stir for 20 to 30 seconds or until the spinach is partially wilted.

5. Pour the eggs into the skillet and stir for 2 minutes or until the eggs are fluffy and scrambled.

6. Transfer to a plate, season with salt and pepper, and serve.

Variation Tip: Switch up next week's breakfast by adding your creative twist on the ingredients in this recipe. Great additions include tomatoes, kale, chard, broccoli, leeks, and asparagus.

PER SERVING CALORIES: 330; TOTAL FAT: 26G; SATURATED FAT: 8G; PROTEIN: 2G; TOTAL CARBOHYDRATES: 12G; FIBER: 2G; CHOLESTEROL: 414MG; MACROS: FAT: 71%; PROTEIN: 2%; CARBS: 27%

MUSHROOM AND CHIVE OMELET

EASY, NUT-FREE, QUICK PREP, UNDER 30 MINUTES

SERVES 1 | PREP TIME: **5 MINUTES** | COOK TIME: **5 MINUTES**

I love mushrooms, and they get the chance to shine in this light and refreshing omelet that combines a deep flavor and meaty texture with fresh chives for a perfect bite.

1 tablespoon avocado oil

2 large eggs

1 garlic clove, minced

1 tablespoon finely chopped white onion

¼ cup finely chopped mushrooms

1 tablespoon finely chopped fresh chives

Sea salt

Freshly ground black pepper

1. Heat the avocado oil in an 8-inch skillet over medium-high heat for 3 minutes or until the oil starts to shimmer.

2. In a small bowl, whisk the eggs.

3. Sauté the garlic and onion for 1 to 2 minutes or until softened.

4. Add the mushrooms and chives and cook for an additional minute or until the mushrooms are brown.

5. Add the eggs and gently tilt the skillet back and forth until the eggs coat the pan evenly.

6. Season with salt and pepper.

7. Cook for 2 minutes or until the eggs are no longer visibly runny.

8. Carefully flip the eggs with a spatula without breaking them and cook for an additional 2 minutes or until firm.

9. Transfer to a plate and fold in half before serving.

Variation Tip: If you can't find fresh chives, use fresh leeks or scallions instead.

PER SERVING CALORIES: 284; TOTAL FAT: 24G; SATURATED FAT: 5G; PROTEIN: 14G; TOTAL CARBOHYDRATES: 3G; FIBER: 1G; CHOLESTEROL: 372MG; MACROS: FAT: 76%; PROTEIN: 20%; CARBS: 4%

SUNRISE EGGS OVER HAM

5 INGREDIENTS OR FEWER, EASY, NUT-FREE, QUICK PREP, UNDER 30 MINUTES

SERVES 4 | PREP TIME: **5 MINUTES** | COOK TIME: **10 MINUTES**

Enjoy delicious pan-seared ham under a perfectly fried sunny-side up egg.

4 slices nitrate- and
   sugar-free ham

2 tablespoons avocado oil

4 large eggs

Sea salt

Freshly ground black pepper

1. Heat the ham in a large skillet over medium-high heat for 5 minutes or until it starts to brown.

2. Carefully flip the ham with a spatula and cook for an additional 2 minutes or until browned. Transfer to a plate and return the skillet to the burner.

3. Heat the avocado oil over medium-high heat for 3 minutes or until the oil starts to shimmer.

4. Crack the eggs, one at a time, into the heated skillet and cover.

5. Leave the eggs undisturbed for 2 minutes or until the whites have set but the yolks are still runny.

6. Carefully remove the eggs and place one atop each ham slice.

7. Season with salt and pepper and serve.

Variation Tip: Use leftover Honey-Orange Glazed Ham (page 157) for this recipe.

PER SERVING CALORIES: 178; TOTAL FAT: 14G; SATURATED FAT: 3G; PROTEIN: 11G; TOTAL CARBOHYDRATES: 2G; FIBER: 0G; CHOLESTEROL: 202MG; MACROS: FAT: 71%; PROTEIN: 25%; CARBS: 4%

SAUSAGE AND SPINACH EGG MUFFINS

MAKES 12 MUFFINS | PREP TIME: **5 MINUTES** | COOK TIME: **30 MINUTES**
This easy-to-assemble, mess-free meal is great for busy people and families.

8 large eggs

½ cup full-fat coconut milk

4 fully cooked breakfast sausages, cut into ¼-inch pieces

1 cup chopped spinach

¼ cup chopped scallions, white and green parts

2 medium garlic cloves, minced

Sea salt

Freshly ground black pepper

1. Preheat the oven to 350°F. Line a muffin tin with paper liners or lightly grease with avocado oil.

2. In a large bowl, whisk together the eggs and coconut milk.

3. Fold in the sausage, spinach, scallions, and garlic.

4. Season with salt and pepper.

5. Fill each muffin cup two-thirds full.

6. Bake for 30 to 35 minutes or until the middle is set and the eggs are no longer visibly runny.

7. Remove from the oven and cool in the pan before serving.

Variation Tip: To add vibrant flavor, use Fresh Herbed Breakfast Sausages (page 59) for this recipe.

PER SERVING (1 MUFFIN) CALORIES: 162; TOTAL FAT: 14G; SATURATED FAT: 6G; PROTEIN: 7G; TOTAL CARBOHYDRATES: 2G; FIBER: 0G; CHOLESTEROL: 139MG; MACROS: FAT: 78%; PROTEIN: 17%; CARBS: 5%

SPINACH AND EGG STUFFED PEPPERS

EASY, NUT-FREE, QUICK PREP

SERVES 4 | PREP TIME: 5 MINUTES | COOK TIME: 30 MINUTES

Elevate your breakfast game with these fun egg-and-veggie-stuffed peppers!

2 bell peppers, tops removed and seeded

6 large eggs

1 cup chopped spinach

2 tablespoons chopped sun-dried tomatoes

2 tablespoons finely chopped black olives

1½ teaspoons finely chopped fresh chives

Sea salt

Freshly ground black pepper

1. Preheat the oven to 400°F.

2. Place each pepper into a compartment in a muffin tin.

3. In a medium bowl, whisk the eggs.

4. Fold in the spinach, sun-dried tomatoes, olives, and chives.

5. Season with salt and pepper.

6. Fill each pepper two-thirds full and bake for 30 minutes or until the eggs are golden and firm to the touch. Let stand for 5 minutes before serving.

Variation Tip: Switch up next week's breakfast by adding your creative twist on the ingredients in this recipe.

PER SERVING CALORIES: 144; TOTAL FAT: 8G; SATURATED FAT: 2G; PROTEIN: 11G; TOTAL CARBOHYDRATES: 7G; FIBER: 1G; CHOLESTEROL: 279MG; MACROS: FAT: 50%; PROTEIN: 31%; CARBS: 19%

AVOCADO EGG TANKERS

SERVES 2 | PREP TIME: 5 MINUTES | COOK TIME: 20 MINUTES

Loaded with healthy fats, proteins, and flavor, this recipe is fit for a satisfying breakfast or snack on any day of the week.

---

1 large avocado,
    halved lengthwise

2 medium eggs

Sea salt

Freshly ground black pepper

1. Preheat the oven to 425°F.

2. Using a tablespoon, remove 1 to 2 tablespoons of the green flesh of each avocado half or enough to create a well that will fit a medium egg.

3. Place each avocado half into a compartment in a muffin tin. (This will prevent the avocado from spilling the egg.)

4. Crack 1 egg into each avocado half.

5. Season with salt and pepper.

6. Carefully place the muffin tin in the oven and bake for 20 minutes or until the egg white is completely set and no longer runny. Let stand for 5 minutes before serving.

> **Ingredient Tip:** To amp up the flavor, top with bacon bits, chives, hot sauce, or scallions.

PER SERVING CALORIES: 222; TOTAL FAT: 18G; SATURATED FAT: 3G; PROTEIN: 7G; TOTAL CARBOHYDRATES: 8G; FIBER: 6G; CHOLESTEROL: 164MG; MACROS: FAT: 73%; PROTEIN: 13%; CARBS: 14%

GOOD MORNING NACHOS

EASY, NUT-FREE, QUICK PREP, UNDER 30 MINUTES

SERVES 2 | PREP TIME: 10 MINUTES | COOK TIME: 10 MINUTES

This recipe uses a sweet and spicy base topped with runny yolks, fresh pico de gallo, and creamy avocado to put a twist on nachos, making them a delicious breakfast dish.

FOR THE PICO DE GALLO

⅔ cup chopped Roma tomatoes

½ cup finely chopped red onion

½ medium jalapeño, chopped (optional)

2 tablespoons freshly squeezed lime juice

¼ cup finely chopped fresh cilantro

¼ teaspoon sea salt

FOR THE NACHOS

2 tablespoons avocado oil, divided

1 small sweet potato, peeled and cut into ¼-inch pieces

1 tablespoon Two-Minute Taco Seasoning (page 231)

2 large eggs

½ medium avocado, sliced

TO MAKE THE PICO DE GALLO

In a medium bowl, combine the tomatoes, onion, jalapeño (if using), lime juice, cilantro, and salt. Set aside to marinate.

TO MAKE THE NACHOS

1. Heat 1 tablespoon of avocado oil in a large skillet over medium-high heat for 3 minutes or until the oil starts to shimmer.

2. Cook the sweet potato for 5 to 7 minutes or until fork-tender.

3. Add the taco seasoning and stir until the sweet potato is evenly coated. Transfer the sweet potato to a plate and return the skillet to the burner.

4. Heat the remaining 1 tablespoon of avocado oil over medium-high heat for 3 minutes or until the oil starts to shimmer.

5. Crack the eggs into the heated skillet and cover. Let the eggs cook undisturbed for 2 minutes or until the whites are set but the yolks are still runny.

6. Place the eggs onto the sweet potato and top with the pico de gallo and avocado.

> Ingredient Tip: Save time by preparing the pico de gallo and taco seasoning the night before.

PER SERVING CALORIES: 366; TOTAL FAT: 26G; SATURATED FAT: 4G; PROTEIN: 9G; TOTAL CARBOHYDRATES: 24G; FIBER: 6G; CHOLESTEROL: 186MG; MACROS: FAT: 64%; PROTEIN: 12%; CARBS: 24%

BACON AND EGG BREAKFAST BURRITO

5 INGREDIENTS OR FEWER, EASY, QUICK PREP, UNDER 30 MINUTES

SERVES 1 | PREP TIME: 5 MINUTES | COOK TIME: 10 MINUTES

Traditional breakfast burritos are filled with American classics. In this one, you can enjoy the saltiness of bacon and the creaminess of scrambled eggs married together in a sweet coconut wrap.

2 large eggs

2 nitrate- and sugar-free bacon slices

1 tablespoon finely chopped white onion

1 tablespoon chopped spinach

1 coconut wrap

1. In a small bowl, whisk the eggs. Set aside.

2. Heat the bacon in an 8-inch skillet over medium-high heat for 5 minutes or until the bacon is crisp and brown.

3. Remove the bacon from the skillet and put it onto a paper towel–lined plate to remove excess grease.

4. Return the skillet with the bacon grease to the burner, and sauté the onion for 1 to 2 minutes or until softened.

5. Add the spinach and stir for 20 to 30 seconds or until the spinach is slightly wilted.

6. Pour the eggs into the skillet and stir for 2 minutes or until they are fluffy and scrambled.

7. Place the eggs and vegetables onto a coconut wrap, top with the bacon, and roll into a burrito.

Variation Tip: If you're unable to find coconut wraps at your local health food grocer, make AIP/Allergen-Free Tortillas (page 36).

PER SERVING CALORIES: 400; TOTAL FAT: 28G; SATURATED FAT: 8G; PROTEIN: 27G; TOTAL CARBOHYDRATES: 10G; FIBER: 1G; CHOLESTEROL: 414MG; MACROS: FAT: 63%; PROTEIN: 27%; CARBS: 10%

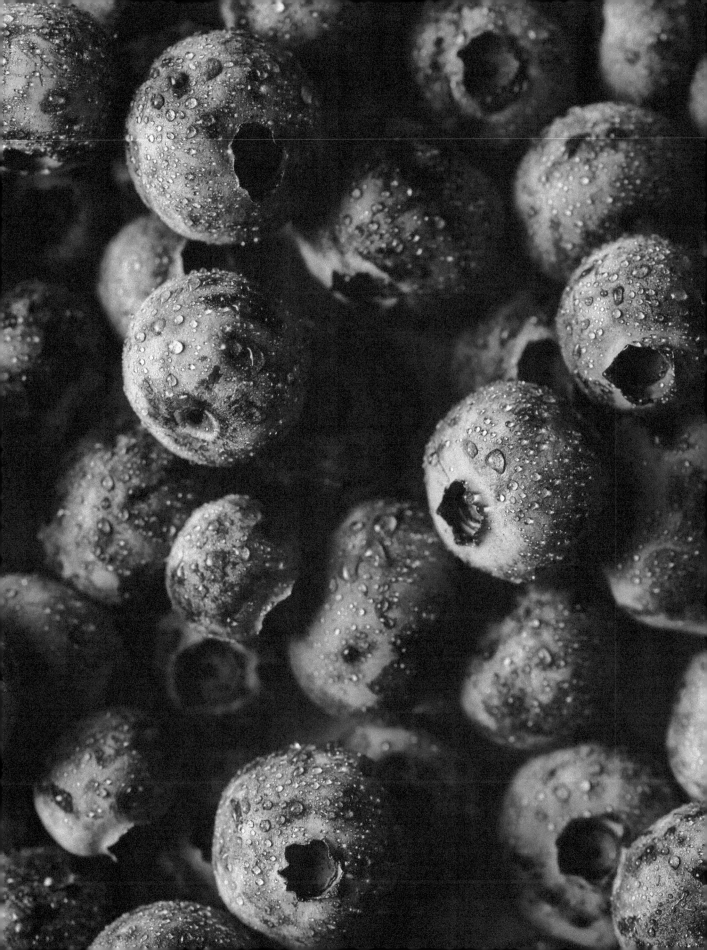

CHAPTER FIVE

EGGLESS AIP/ ALLERGEN- FREE BREAKFASTS

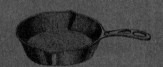

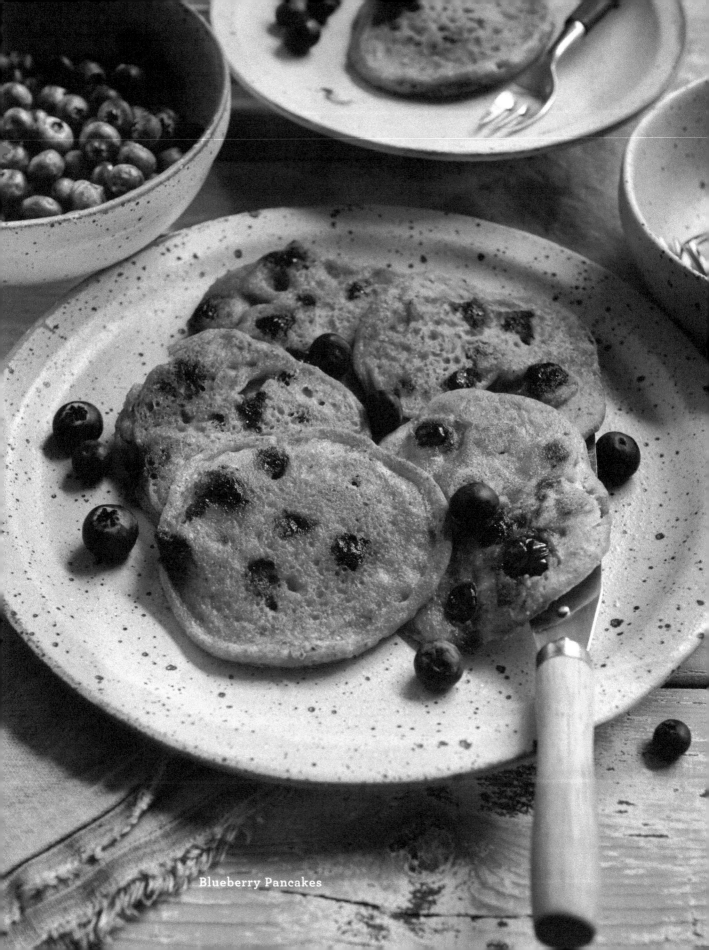

Blueberry Pancakes

BLUEBERRY PANCAKES

AIP-FRIENDLY, ALLERGEN-FREE, EGG-FREE, QUICK PREP, UNDER 30 MINUTES

SERVES 6 | PREP TIME: **5 MINUTES** | COOK TIME: **10 MINUTES**

Blueberry pancakes made with tigernut flour guarantee a fluffy, nutty-flavored, and fiber-enriched breakfast.

2 tablespoons coconut oil

1 cup full-fat coconut milk, more if needed

1 tablespoon unflavored gelatin powder

¾ cup tigernut flour

¼ cup arrowroot flour

¼ teaspoon sea salt

½ cup blueberries

1. Heat the coconut oil in a large skillet over medium-high heat (or 375°F if using a pancake griddle) for 3 minutes or until the oil starts to shimmer.

2. In a large bowl, whisk together the coconut milk, gelatin powder, tigernut flour, arrowroot flour, and salt. If the batter seems too thick, add extra coconut milk, 1 tablespoon at a time, until it reaches the desired consistency.

3. Fold in the blueberries.

4. Pour or scoop ¼ cup of batter onto the skillet for each pancake.

5. Fry for 2 to 3 minutes per side or until golden brown.

> Variation Tip: Switch up next week's breakfast by adding your favorite fruit or seasoning. Great options include peaches, strawberries, or pumpkin spice.

PER SERVING CALORIES: 242; TOTAL FAT: 18G; SATURATED FAT: 13G; PROTEIN: 6G; TOTAL CARBOHYDRATES: 14G; FIBER: 6G; CHOLESTEROL: 0MG; MACROS: FAT: 67%; PROTEIN: 10%; CARBS: 23%

SWEET POTATO HASH BROWNS

AIP-FRIENDLY, ALLERGEN-FREE, EASY, EGG-FREE, UNDER 30 MINUTES

SERVES 4 | PREP TIME: **10 MINUTES** | COOK TIME: **5 MINUTES**

Crisp and crunchy sweet potato hash browns are an excellent addition to any breakfast or brunch.

3 cups peeled shredded
   sweet potatoes (about
   2 medium
   sweet potatoes)

2 tablespoons coconut oil

1 tablespoon arrowroot flour

½ teaspoon sea salt

1 teaspoon freshly ground
   black pepper

1. Wrap the sweet potatoes in a paper towel and squeeze to remove any excess moisture.

2. Heat the coconut oil in a cast iron skillet over medium-high heat for 3 minutes or until the oil starts to shimmer.

3. In a medium bowl, combine the sweet potatoes, arrowroot flour, salt, and pepper.

4. Gently scoop 2 tablespoons of the mixture at a time into the skillet and flatten with a spatula.

5. Fry each hash brown for 2 to 3 minutes or until golden and crispy. Flip and fry for an additional 2 to 3 minutes or until crisp and cooked through.

6. Remove the hash browns from the skillet and put onto a paper towel–lined plate to remove excess oil.

Make-Ahead Tip: Shred the sweet potatoes in advance with a cheese grater, mandoline, or food processor.

PER SERVING CALORIES: 123; TOTAL FAT: 7G; SATURATED FAT: 6G; PROTEIN: 1G; TOTAL CARBOHYDRATES: 14G; FIBER: 2G; CHOLESTEROL: 0MG; MACROS: FAT: 51%; PROTEIN: 5%; CARBS: 44%

FRESH HERBED BREAKFAST SAUSAGES

AIP-FRIENDLY, ALLERGEN-FREE, EASY, EGG-FREE, QUICK PREP, UNDER 30 MINUTES

SERVES 4 | PREP TIME: 5 MINUTES | COOK TIME: 10 MINUTES

Enjoy these fresh and easy-to-make breakfast sausages with any meal. They're made with minimal ingredients and no additives, so eat one or a few!

---

1 tablespoon coconut oil

1 pound ground pork

2 teaspoons dried thyme

2 teaspoons dried sage

1 teaspoon sea salt

½ teaspoon garlic powder

½ teaspoon onion powder

1. Heat the coconut oil in a cast iron skillet over medium-high heat for 3 minutes or until the oil starts to shimmer.

2. In a medium bowl, combine the pork, thyme, sage, salt, garlic powder, and onion powder.

3. Divide the meat into 8 to 10 (2-inch) balls, using your hands to press each into a patty.

4. Fry the patties for 5 minutes per side or until the outer layer is crisp and the internal temperature reaches 160°F. Serve immediately.

> **Variation Tip:** Switch up the spice profile by adding rosemary, chives, oregano, or basil.

PER SERVING CALORIES: 264; TOTAL FAT: 20G; SATURATED FAT: 9G; PROTEIN: 20G; TOTAL CARBOHYDRATES: 1G; FIBER: 0G; CHOLESTEROL: 75MG; MACROS: FAT: 68%; PROTEIN: 30%; CARBS: 2%

SWEET POTATO TOAST

5 INGREDIENTS OR FEWER, AIP-FRIENDLY, ALLERGEN-FREE, EASY, EGG-FREE, QUICK PREP,
UNDER 30 MINUTES

SERVES 4 | PREP TIME: 5 MINUTES | COOK TIME: 15 MINUTES

Sweet potato toast is an excellent addition to any breakfast, as its sweetness provides an experience standard bread cannot duplicate.

1 large sweet potato, peeled

2 tablespoons melted
    coconut oil

Sea salt

Freshly ground black pepper

Homemade jam, for topping

1. Preheat the oven to 425°F. Top a baking sheet with an oven-safe wire rack.

2. Using a mandoline or knife, carefully cut the sweet potato into ⅛-inch-thick slices.

3. Brush both sides of each slice with the coconut oil and place onto the prepared rack.

4. Season with salt and pepper.

5. Bake the sweet potato slices for 12 minutes or until the edges start to brown.

6. Remove from the oven and top with the jam. Serve immediately.

Storage Tip: Store sweet potato toast in the refrigerator between parchment paper or wax paper in an airtight container. When you're ready to eat them, toast them on low in a toaster oven for 1 to 2 minutes.

PER SERVING CALORIES: 95; TOTAL FAT: 7G; SATURATED FAT: 6G;
PROTEIN: 1G; TOTAL CARBOHYDRATES: 7G; FIBER: 1G;
CHOLESTEROL: 0MG; MACROS: FAT: 66%; PROTEIN: 4%; CARBS: 30%

BANANA CREAM PIE PARFAIT

AIP-FRIENDLY, ALLERGEN-FREE, EGG-FREE

SERVES 4 | PREP TIME: 15 MINUTES, PLUS 1 HOUR TO CHILL | COOK TIME: 15 MINUTES
Indulge in layers of sweet banana flavor, smooth pudding, and cookie crunch with this tempting morning start!

FOR THE PUDDING

1 (13.5-ounce) can full-fat coconut milk

1 tablespoon unflavored gelatin powder

3 large bananas, divided

1 teaspoon pure maple syrup

¼ teaspoon sea salt

FOR THE PIE CRUMBLE

½ cup coconut flour

¼ cup unsweetened shredded coconut

4 tablespoons coconut oil

1 tablespoon pure maple syrup

¼ teaspoon ground cinnamon

¼ teaspoon sea salt

TO MAKE THE PUDDING

1. In a medium bowl, whisk together the coconut milk and gelatin. Set aside for 15 minutes to thicken.

2. Pour the mixture into a blender. Add 2 bananas, maple syrup, and sea salt. Blend on high speed for 30 seconds or until smooth with no visible banana chunks.

3. Pour the pudding into an airtight container and set in the refrigerator for 1 hour or until the pudding is firm.

TO MAKE THE PIE CRUMBLE

1. Preheat the oven to 350°F. Line an edged baking sheet with parchment paper.

2. In a food processor, pulse the coconut flour, shredded coconut, coconut oil, maple syrup, cinnamon, and salt 10 to 20 times or until combined but still crumbly.

3. Pour the pie crumble onto the prepared baking sheet and bake for 12 minutes or until golden brown.

4. Slice the remaining banana.

5. To assemble the parfait, layer an 8-ounce mason jar with the pie crumble, then a few slices of banana, followed by a layer of pudding. Repeat until full, then continue with three more jars. Served chilled.

> **Variation Tip:** Maple syrup can be swapped out for raw honey in both the pudding and crumble.

PER SERVING CALORIES: 668; TOTAL FAT: 48G; SATURATED FAT: 41G; PROTEIN: 11G; TOTAL CARBOHYDRATES: 48G; FIBER: 19G; CHOLESTEROL: 0MG; MACROS: FAT: 65%; PROTEIN: 6%; CARBS: 29%

AIP GRANOLA BARS

AIP-FRIENDLY, ALLERGEN-FREE, EASY, EGG-FREE

MAKES 9 BARS | PREP TIME: 10 MINUTES, PLUS 3 HOURS TO SET

You will not find any tree nuts here! Despite their name, tigernuts are a fiber-rich tuber. They give these granola bars a nutty flavor.

8 Medjool dates, pitted and chopped

2 cups sliced tigernuts

1 cup unsweetened shredded coconut

⅓ cup melted coconut oil

2 tablespoons pure maple syrup

4 tablespoons collagen powder

1 teaspoon ground cinnamon

1. Line an 8-by-8-inch baking dish with parchment paper or wax paper.

2. In a food processor, blend the dates, tigernuts, and coconut on high speed for 10 to 15 seconds or until well combined yet chunky.

3. Transfer the contents to a large bowl and combine with the coconut oil, maple syrup, collagen powder, and cinnamon.

4. Pour the granola into the prepared dish and flatten it with a lightly greased spatula (or your hands).

5. Set in the refrigerator for 3 hours or until hardened.

6. Remove the parchment paper and cut into 9 bars.

Variation Tip: For a twist on this recipe, fold in ¼ cup of dried apples, blueberries, or cherries during step 3.

PER SERVING (1 BAR) CALORIES: 338; TOTAL FAT: 18G; SATURATED FAT: 14G; PROTEIN: 5G; TOTAL CARBOHYDRATES: 39G; FIBER: 7G; CHOLESTEROL: 0MG; MACROS: FAT: 48%; PROTEIN: 6%; CARBS: 46%

SUNRISE BREAKFAST HASH

AIP-FRIENDLY, ALLERGEN-FREE, EASY, EGG-FREE, QUICK PREP, UNDER 30 MINUTES

SERVES 4 | PREP TIME: **5 MINUTES** | COOK TIME: **15 MINUTES**

Who said breakfast has to consist solely of breakfast foods? Relish the sweetness of the sweet potatoes and savor the beef's earthiness in this perfectly seasoned sunrise hash.

2 tablespoons coconut oil

1 large sweet potato, peeled and cut into ¼-inch pieces

1 medium white onion, chopped

1 pound 80/20 ground beef

2 teaspoons garlic powder

2 teaspoons onion powder

1 teaspoon sea salt

1. Heat the coconut oil in a cast iron skillet over medium-high heat for 3 minutes or until the oil starts to shimmer.

2. Add the sweet potato and onion and cook for 8 minutes or until the sweet potato is fork-tender and the onion is translucent.

3. Transfer the mixture to a large bowl.

4. Return the skillet to the burner and add the ground beef, cooking over medium-high heat for 5 minutes or until browned.

5. Drain any excess grease, then stir in the garlic powder, onion powder, and salt.

6. Return the vegetables to the skillet, stir to combine, and serve.

> **Variation Tip:** Instead of ground beef, use ground turkey or pork.

PER SERVING CALORIES: 370; TOTAL FAT: 26G; SATURATED FAT: 26G; PROTEIN: 23G; TOTAL CARBOHYDRATES: 11G; FIBER: 2G; CHOLESTEROL: 59MG; MACROS: FAT: 63%; PROTEIN: 25%; CARBS: 12%

APPLE-CINNAMON PORRIDGE

AIP-FRIENDLY, ALLERGEN-FREE, EASY, EGG-FREE, QUICK PREP, UNDER 30 MINUTES

SERVES 4 | PREP TIME: 5 MINUTES | COOK TIME: 20 MINUTES

My two favorite flavors combine here to give you an autumnal breakfast that's perfect for any day of the year. Savor the sweet notes of the apples and the spice of the cinnamon in every bite.

2 cups full-fat coconut milk

½ cup Grated Cauliflower Rice (page 37)

½ cup shredded coconut

2 apples, grated

1 tablespoon pure maple syrup

1 teaspoon ground cinnamon

1. In a medium saucepan, combine the coconut milk, cauliflower rice, coconut, apples, maple syrup, and cinnamon over medium heat. Bring to a gentle boil, cover, and simmer for 20 minutes or until the porridge is tender and fragrant.

2. Remove from the heat and serve immediately.

> **Variation Tip:** Top with additional apples, raisins, or a drizzle of maple syrup to enhance your porridge.

PER SERVING CALORIES: 416; TOTAL FAT: 32G; SATURATED FAT: 28G; PROTEIN: 4G; TOTAL CARBOHYDRATES: 28G; FIBER: 7G; CHOLESTEROL: 0MG; MACROS: FAT: 69%; PROTEIN: 4%; CARBS: 27%

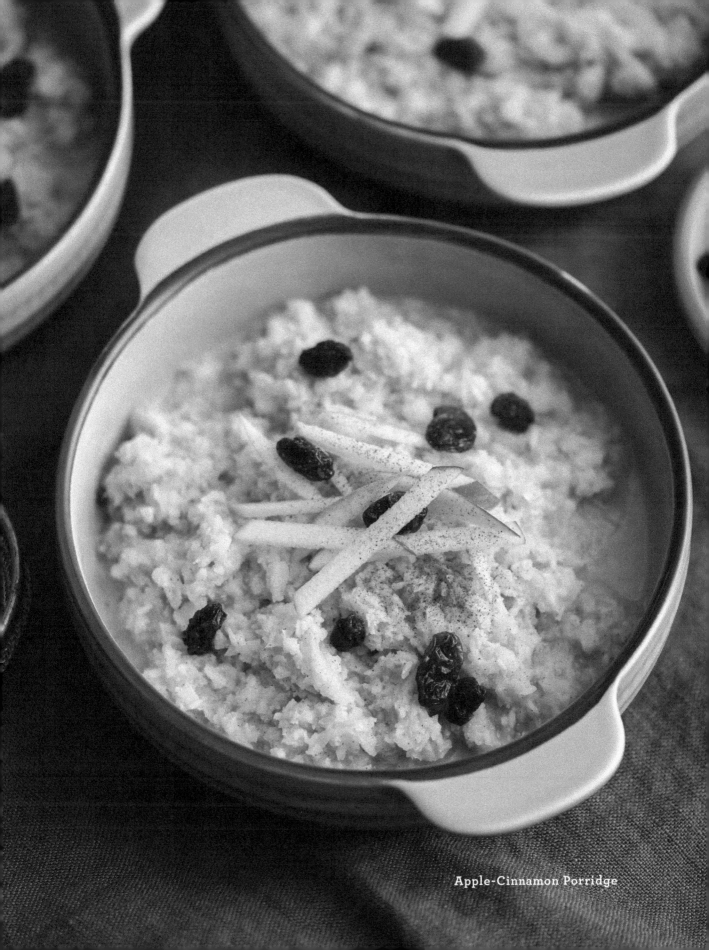

Apple-Cinnamon Porridge

CASSAVA WAFFLES

AIP-FRIENDLY, ALLERGEN-FREE, EGG-FREE, QUICK PREP, UNDER 30 MINUTES

MAKES 4 WAFFLES | PREP TIME: **5 MINUTES** | COOK TIME: **5 MINUTES**

These cassava waffles will make a delicious addition to your breakfast table and are perfect for those who are following the autoimmune protocol or have allergies.

Coconut oil cooking spray

1 cup cassava flour

¼ teaspoon baking soda

¼ teaspoon sea salt

1 cup full-fat coconut milk, more if needed

1 tablespoon melted coconut oil

1. Preheat a waffle iron and lightly grease both sides with cooking spray.

2. In a medium bowl, combine the cassava flour, baking soda, and salt.

3. Whisk in the coconut milk and coconut oil. If the batter seems too thick, add extra coconut milk, 1 tablespoon at a time, until it reaches the desired consistency.

4. Fill the waffle iron, close, and bake for 5 minutes or until the waffles are cooked and crispy. Serve immediately.

Variation Tip: During step 3, fold in your favorite fresh fruit or add a sprinkle of cinnamon or pumpkin spice.

PER SERVING (1 WAFFLE) CALORIES: 294; TOTAL FAT: 18G; SATURATED FAT: 16G; PROTEIN: 2G; TOTAL CARBOHYDRATES: 31G; FIBER: 6G; CHOLESTEROL: 0MG; MACROS: FAT: 55%; PROTEIN: 3%; CARBS: 42%

VERY BERRY PARFAIT

AIP-FRIENDLY, ALLERGEN-FREE, EGG-FREE, QUICK PREP

SERVES 4 | PREP TIME: 20 MINUTES, PLUS 1 HOUR TO CHILL

Entice your taste buds with a coconut base pudding that has layers of sweet berries and a toothsome crunch.

FOR THE PUDDING

- 1 (13.5-ounce) can full-fat coconut milk
- 2 tablespoons raw honey
- 2 teaspoons unflavored gelatin powder

FOR THE PARFAIT LAYERS

- 1 cup nut- and seed-free paleo-approved granola
- 1 cup chopped fresh strawberries
- 1 cup fresh blueberries

TO MAKE THE PUDDING

In a medium bowl, whisk together the coconut milk, honey, and gelatin until well combined. Set aside for 15 minutes to thicken.

TO MAKE THE PARFAIT LAYERS

1. To assemble the parfait, layer an 8-ounce mason jar with the granola, strawberries, blueberries, and a layer of pudding. Repeat until full, then continue with three more jars.

2. Refrigerate for at least 1 hour before serving.

> **Variation Tip:** For new and exciting flavors, use fruits such as bananas, pineapples, mangos, or my favorite, cherries.

PER SERVING CALORIES: 476; TOTAL FAT: 32G; SATURATED FAT: 21G; PROTEIN: 13G; TOTAL CARBOHYDRATES: 34G; FIBER: 15G; CHOLESTEROL: 0MG; MACROS: FAT: 61%; PROTEIN: 11%; CARBS: 28%

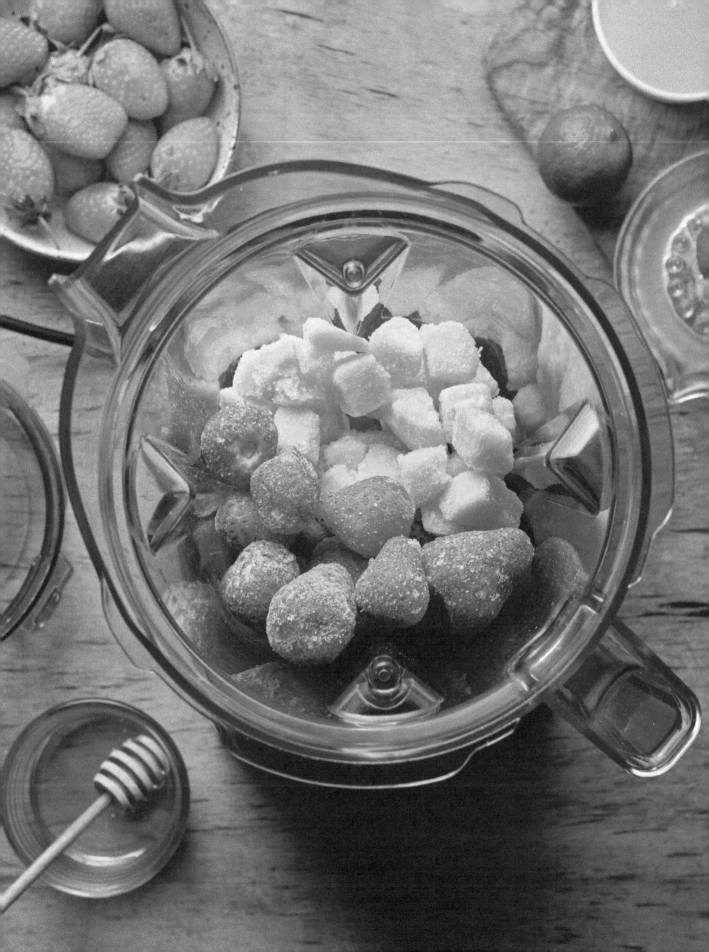

CHAPTER SIX

BEVERAGES AND SMOOTHIES

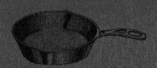

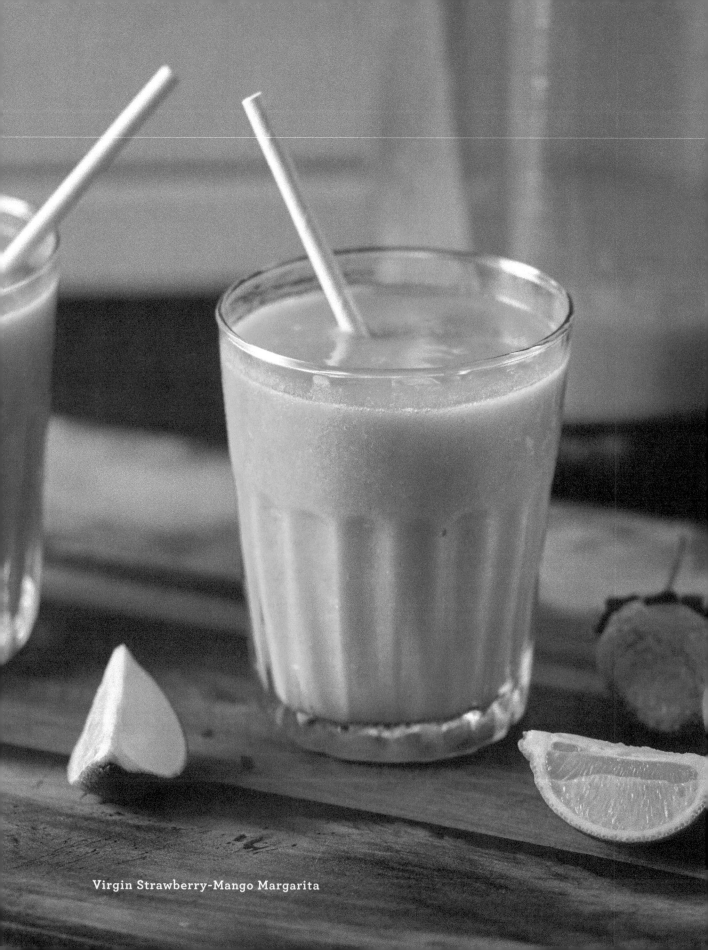

Virgin Strawberry-Mango Margarita

VIRGIN STRAWBERRY-MANGO MARGARITA

5 INGREDIENTS OR FEWER, AIP-FRIENDLY, ALLERGEN-FREE, EASY, EGG-FREE, NUT-FREE, QUICK PREP, UNDER 30 MINUTES

SERVES 1 | PREP TIME: 5 MINUTES

This beverage is a sweet treat and a fun addition to any party or event.

½ cup frozen strawberries

½ cup frozen mangos

1½ cups orange juice

1 tablespoon freshly squeezed lime juice

1 tablespoon raw honey

In a blender, add the strawberries, mangos, orange and lime juices, and honey. Blend on high for 1 minute or until the fruit is evenly and smoothly blended.

Variation Tip: Other great fruit options for these virgin margaritas include pineapple, blueberries, banana, and peaches.

PER SERVING CALORIES: 325; TOTAL FAT: 1G; SATURATED FAT: 0G; PROTEIN: 4G; TOTAL CARBOHYDRATES: 75G; FIBER: 4G; CHOLESTEROL: 0MG; MACROS: FAT: 3%; PROTEIN: 5%; CARBS: 92%

BULLETPROOF COFFEE

SERVES 1 | PREP TIME: 5 MINUTES

Bulletproof coffee is an excellent source of saturated fats that will provide your brain with everything it needs to keep you going while leaving you feeling fuller longer.

8 ounces hot coffee

1 tablespoon MCT (medium-chain triglyceride) oil

1 tablespoon ghee

Pinch ground cinnamon

Pinch sea salt

1. In a blender, blend the coffee, MCT oil, and ghee on high for 20 to 30 seconds or until smooth.

2. Serve immediately with a pinch of cinnamon and salt to enhance the flavor.

> Variation Tip: If you can handle small amounts of dairy, swap out ghee for grass-fed butter.

PER SERVING CALORIES: 252; TOTAL FAT: 28G; SATURATED FAT: 23G; PROTEIN: 0G; TOTAL CARBOHYDRATES: 0G; FIBER: 0G; CHOLESTEROL: 35MG; MACROS: FAT: 97%; PROTEIN: 2%; CARBS: 1%

PUMPKIN SPICE LATTE

5 INGREDIENTS OR FEWER, ALLERGEN-FREE, EASY, EGG-FREE, QUICK PREP, UNDER 30 MINUTES

SERVES 1 | PREP TIME: 5 MINUTES

Ditch tomorrow's coffee run and make this smooth and flavorful pumpkin spice latte instead. Treat yourself and top it with cinnamon and chopped walnuts if you like.

8 ounces hot coffee

½ cup full-fat coconut milk

4 tablespoons pumpkin purée

1 tablespoon raw honey

½ teaspoon vanilla extract

1. In a blender, blend the coffee, coconut milk, pumpkin purée, honey, and vanilla on high for 30 to 45 seconds or until smooth.

2. Serve immediately.

> **Variation Tip:** Try this recipe with almond milk instead of coconut milk for a nutty flavor.

PER SERVING CALORIES: 393; TOTAL FAT: 29G; SATURATED FAT: 26G; PROTEIN: 4G; TOTAL CARBOHYDRATES: 29G; FIBER: 5G; CHOLESTEROL: 0MG; MACROS: FAT: 66%; PROTEIN: 4%; CARBS: 30%

FRENCH VANILLA COFFEE CREAMER

AIP-FRIENDLY, ALLERGEN-FREE, EGG-FREE, QUICK PREP, UNDER 30 MINUTES

SERVES 6 | PREP TIME: 5 MINUTES

Lighten up your coffee with this delicious dairy-free coffee creamer that's full of sweet vanilla flavor.

1 (13.5-ounce) can full-fat coconut milk

2 tablespoons pure maple syrup

2 teaspoons vanilla extract

Pour the coconut milk, maple syrup, and vanilla into a sealable pint jar, cover, and shake for 1 to 2 minutes or until ingredients are evenly combined.

Storage Tip: Store the coffee creamer in the sealable pint-size jar in the refrigerator for 7 to 10 days.

PER SERVING (2 TABLESPOONS) CALORIES: 175; TOTAL FAT: 15G; SATURATED FAT: 14G; PROTEIN: 2G; TOTAL CARBOHYDRATES: 8G; FIBER: 1G; CHOLESTEROL: 0MG; MACROS: FAT: 77%; PROTEIN: 5%; CARBS: 18%

COCONUT AND AVOCADO SMOOTHIE

5 INGREDIENTS OR FEWER, AIP-FRIENDLY, ALLERGEN-FREE, EASY, EGG-FREE, QUICK PREP, UNDER 30 MINUTES

SERVES 2 | PREP TIME: 5 MINUTES

This nutrient-dense and coconut-packed smoothie is perfect for a quick morning breakfast or a post-workout snack.

1 medium avocado

½ cup full-fat coconut milk

½ cup unsweetened coconut yogurt

½ cup coconut cream

8 ice cubes

1. In a blender, blend the avocado, coconut milk, yogurt, coconut cream, and ice cubes on high speed for 30 to 60 seconds or until smooth.

2. Serve immediately.

> **Storage Tip:** Make ahead and store in the freezer for 24 hours. Although the smoothie can be stored for longer, the avocado will likely oxidize beyond 24 hours' storage time.

PER SERVING CALORIES: 521; TOTAL FAT: 41G; SATURATED FAT: 27G; PROTEIN: 4G; TOTAL CARBOHYDRATES: 34G; FIBER: 8G; CHOLESTEROL: 0MG; MACROS: FAT: 71%; PROTEIN: 3%; CARBS: 26%

GREEN MACHINE SMOOTHIE

SERVES 1 | PREP TIME: **5 MINUTES**

Get your day started with this nutrient-dense smoothie filled with essential leafy greens and delicious sweet fruits.

½ cup frozen mango

½ medium banana

½ medium avocado

½ cup roughly
  chopped spinach

½ cup roughly chopped kale

1 cup full-fat coconut milk,
  more if needed

In a blender, blend the mango, banana, avocado, spinach, kale, and coconut milk on high for 2 minutes or until smooth and creamy. (If the consistency seems too thick, add extra coconut milk, 1 tablespoon at a time, until it's smooth and creamy.)

Variation Tip: Coconut milk can be swapped out for an equal amount of almond milk.

PER SERVING CALORIES: 847; TOTAL FAT: 71G; SATURATED FAT: 53G; PROTEIN: 10G; TOTAL CARBOHYDRATES: 42G; FIBER: 15G; CHOLESTEROL: 0MG; MACROS: FAT: 75%; PROTEIN: 5%; CARBS: 20%

BLUEBERRY PIE SMOOTHIE

5 INGREDIENTS OR FEWER, EASY, EGG-FREE, QUICK PREP, UNDER 30 MINUTES

SERVES 1 | PREP TIME: **5 MINUTES**

If you ever wanted pie for breakfast, this smoothie is for you. Take your traditional blueberry pie and turn it into a sweet and nutrient-dense paleo smoothie.

1 cup frozen blueberries

1 cup almond milk

¼ cup unsweetened shredded coconut

2 tablespoons almond butter

¼ teaspoon ground cinnamon

In a blender, blend the blueberries, almond milk, coconut, almond butter, and cinnamon on high for 1 minute or until smooth and creamy.

> **Variation Tip:** Make this an allergen-free smoothie by replacing the almond milk with coconut milk and the almond butter with sunflower butter.

PER SERVING CALORIES: 483; TOTAL FAT: 35G; SATURATED FAT: 13G; PROTEIN: 10G; TOTAL CARBOHYDRATES: 32G; FIBER: 11G; CHOLESTEROL: 0MG; MACROS: FAT: 65%; PROTEIN: 8%; CARBS: 27%

SWEET SPARKLING LEMONADE

AIP-FRIENDLY, ALLERGEN-FREE, EASY, EGG-FREE, NUT-FREE, QUICK PREP, UNDER 30 MINUTES

MAKES 8 CUPS | PREP TIME: **5 MINUTES** | COOK TIME: **5 MINUTES**

This lemonade is a refreshing, sweet, tangy, and bubbly treat. You'll enjoy the tartness of the freshly squeezed lemons playing nicely with the sweetness of the honey.

1 cup freshly squeezed
   lemon juice (about
   4 to 5 large lemons)

½ cup raw honey

6 cups sparkling
   seltzer water

Ice

Lemon slices (optional)

Fresh mint or
   basil (optional)

1. In a medium saucepan, combine the lemon juice and honey over low heat for 5 minutes or until warmed.

2. Whisk the honey until it has completely dissolved, then remove from the heat and stir in the seltzer water.

3. Carefully pour the lemonade into a pitcher and add ice to fill. Serve chilled with lemon slices or a pinch of mint or basil (if using).

> **Variation Tip:** Swap out honey for maple syrup or coconut sugar.

PER SERVING (1 CUP) CALORIES: 72; TOTAL FAT: 0G; SATURATED FAT: 0G; PROTEIN: 0G; TOTAL CARBOHYDRATES: 18G; FIBER: 0G; CHOLESTEROL: 0MG; MACROS: FAT: 97%; PROTEIN: 2%; CARBS: 1%

SPARKLING ICED GREEN TEA AND LEMON

5 INGREDIENTS OR FEWER, AIP-FRIENDLY, ALLERGEN-FREE, EASY, EGG-FREE, NUT-FREE, QUICK PREP, UNDER 30 MINUTES

MAKES 6 CUPS | PREP TIME: **5 MINUTES** | COOK TIME: **5 MINUTES**

This sparkling iced green tea is an excellent healthy substitution for those who are missing their carbonated beverages. Enjoy all the benefits green tea has to offer while getting your carbonation fix!

2 cups water

4 green tea bags
(with caffeine
or caffeine-free)

4 cups sparkling
seltzer water

Ice

Lemon slices

1. In a medium saucepan, bring the water to a boil.

2. Remove the saucepan from the heat, add the tea bags, and steep for 4 minutes.

3. Remove the tea bags and carefully pour the tea into a glass pitcher.

4. Add the seltzer water and fill with ice.

5. Serve chilled with a slice of lemon.

Variation Tip: Save time by heating the water in a glass bowl for 3 minutes in the microwave.

PER SERVING (1 CUP) CALORIES: 0; TOTAL FAT: 0G; SATURATED FAT: 0G; PROTEIN: 0G; TOTAL CARBOHYDRATES: 0G; FIBER: 0G; CHOLESTEROL: 0MG; MACROS: FAT: 0%; PROTEIN: 0%; CARBS: 0%

HOT CHOCOLATE

SERVES 2 | PREP TIME: **5 MINUTES** | COOK TIME: **5 MINUTES**

You can't go wrong with a cup of hot chocolate after a long day of work or sledding. Enjoy subtle hints of vanilla while savoring chocolate creaminess in every sip.

2 cups almond milk

2 tablespoons cacao powder

1 teaspoon vanilla extract

⅛ teaspoon sea salt

½ cup paleo
   chocolate chips

1. In a medium saucepan, bring the almond milk to a gentle boil over medium heat.

2. Whisk in the cacao powder, vanilla, and salt. Reduce the heat to low.

3. Whisk in the chocolate chips until they are completely dissolved.

4. Remove the hot chocolate from the heat and carefully pour into mugs. Serve immediately.

> Variation Tip: Use coconut milk instead of almond milk for a change of pace and to make this an allergen-free drink that the whole family can enjoy.

PER SERVING CALORIES: 280; TOTAL FAT: 16G; SATURATED FAT: 9G; PROTEIN: 5G; TOTAL CARBOHYDRATES: 29G; FIBER: 15G; CHOLESTEROL: 1MG; MACROS: FAT: 51%; PROTEIN: 8%; CARBS: 41%

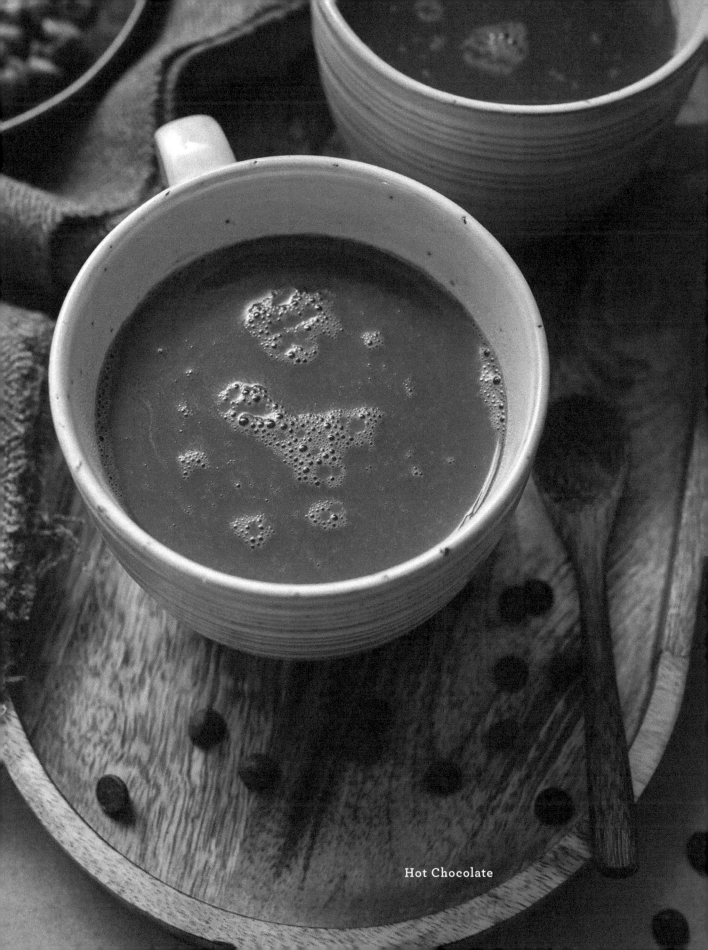

Hot Chocolate

SWEETENED COCONUT WATER

5 INGREDIENTS OR FEWER, AIP-FRIENDLY, ALLERGEN-FREE, EGG-FREE, QUICK PREP, UNDER 30 MINUTES

MAKES 8 CUPS | PREP TIME: **5 MINUTES** | COOK TIME: **5 MINUTES**

Enjoy this refreshing beverage that's full of thirst-quenching coconut flavor and perfect for summertime! When purchasing coconut water, be sure to opt for a pure variety that contains no added fillers or sweeteners.

1 quart water

2 tablespoons raw honey

1 cup pure coconut water
  (or water from
  1 whole coconut)

1. In a medium saucepan, combine the water and honey over low heat until the honey is dissolved, about 5 minutes. Remove the water from the heat and pour it into a glass jug, pitcher, or resealable bottle.

2. Add the coconut water and stir. Serve cold.

Variation Tip: Swap out honey for an equal amount of maple syrup or omit it completely for a sugar-free beverage.

PER SERVING (1 CUP) CALORIES: 20; TOTAL FAT: 0G; SATURATED FAT: 0G; PROTEIN: 0G; TOTAL CARBOHYDRATES: 5G; FIBER: 0G; CHOLESTEROL: 0MG; MACROS: FAT: 1%; PROTEIN: 1%; CARBS: 98%

KOMBUCHA

5 INGREDIENTS OR FEWER, AIP-FRIENDLY, ALLERGEN-FREE, EGG-FREE, NUT-FREE, QUICK PREP

MAKES 16 CUPS | PREP TIME: **5 MINUTES, PLUS 7 DAYS TO FERMENT** | COOK TIME: **10 MINUTES**

Enjoy all the health benefits this legendary fermented tea has to offer! Switch up the flavor profile by adding chopped fruits, herbs, and spices.

3½ quarts water

1 cup pure cane sugar

8 black tea bags

2 cups kombucha starter tea (homemade or store-bought)

1 SCOBY

1. In a large stockpot, bring the water to a boil over medium-high heat. Once the water is boiling, remove from the heat and whisk in the sugar for 1 minute or until the sugar is completely dissolved.

2. Add the tea bags and steep until the water is completely cooled. Remove the tea bags and discard.

3. In the stockpot, combine the kombucha starter tea and the steeped tea and stir for 30 seconds. Pour the contents from the stockpot into a gallon-sized glass container and add the SCOBY.

4. Using 2 or 3 coffee filters, a paper towel, or cheese-cloth, cover the mouth of the container and secure it tightly with a rubber band.

5. Allow the kombucha to ferment for 7 to 10 days at room temperature away from direct sunlight. Kombucha is ready when it reaches the perfect balance between sweetness and tartness.

Ingredient Tip: When purchasing store-bought kombucha starter tea, make sure that it contains sediment and is unflavored, raw, and unpasteurized.

PER SERVING (1 CUP) CALORIES: 15; TOTAL FAT: 0G; SATURATED FAT: 0G; PROTEIN: 0G; TOTAL CARBOHYDRATES: 4G; FIBER: 0G; CHOLESTEROL: 0MG; MACROS: FAT: 0%; PROTEIN: 0%; CARBS: 100%

SPICED APPLE CIDER

SERVES 8 | PREP TIME: 10 MINUTES, PLUS 1 HOUR TO COOL | COOK TIME: 6 HOURS

Enjoy the delicious tartness of the apples and the sweetness of the coconut sugar mixed with the classic spiced combo of cinnamon and nutmeg.

---

10 medium Gala apples, cored and quartered

½ cup coconut sugar

4 (4-inch) cinnamon sticks

4 tablespoons ground nutmeg

Water

1. Combine the apples, coconut sugar, cinnamon sticks, and nutmeg in a 6-quart or larger slow cooker.

2. Fill with enough water to cover.

3. Cover and cook on low for 4 to 6 hours or until the apples are fork-tender.

4. Allow the cider to cool 30 to 60 minutes.

5. Smash the apples in the slow cooker with a wooden spoon or potato masher until they are broken down.

6. Strain the apple cider into a large bowl and transfer to a glass container for serving. Serve warm or cold.

> Ingredient Tip: Make spiced applesauce with the cooked apples. Instead of disposing of them, transfer the apples to a food processor and blend for 1 minute or until smooth.

PER SERVING CALORIES: 68; TOTAL FAT: 0G; SATURATED FAT: 0G; PROTEIN: 1G; TOTAL CARBOHYDRATES: 16G; FIBER: 3G; CHOLESTEROL: 0MG; MACROS: FAT: 96%; PROTEIN: 3%; CARBS: 1%

VERY FRUITY VIRGIN SANGRIA

AIP-FRIENDLY, ALLERGEN-FREE, EASY, EGG-FREE, NUT-FREE, QUICK PREP

SERVES 4 | PREP TIME: 10 MINUTES, PLUS 3 HOURS TO CHILL

Since this refreshingly fruity drink does not contain alcohol, it's an excellent addition for any party or baby shower.

---

1 lemon, sliced

1 lime, sliced

1 orange, sliced

1 apple, sliced

¾ cup apple juice

¾ cup orange juice

1 tablespoon freshly squeezed lemon juice

4 cups sparkling seltzer water

1. In a glass jug, combine the lemon, lime, orange, and apple slices and the apple, orange, and lemon juices.

2. Refrigerate for 3 hours.

3. Before serving, add the seltzer water and stir.

Variation Tip: Have fun with your virgin sangria by replacing the fresh fruits in this recipe with your favorites for new flavor profiles. Good options include mangos, strawberries, pineapple, or blueberries.

PER SERVING CALORIES: 40; TOTAL FAT: 0G; SATURATED FAT: 0G; PROTEIN: 0G; TOTAL CARBOHYDRATES: 10G; FIBER: 0G; CHOLESTEROL: 0MG; MACROS: FAT: 97%; PROTEIN: 2%; CARBS: 1%

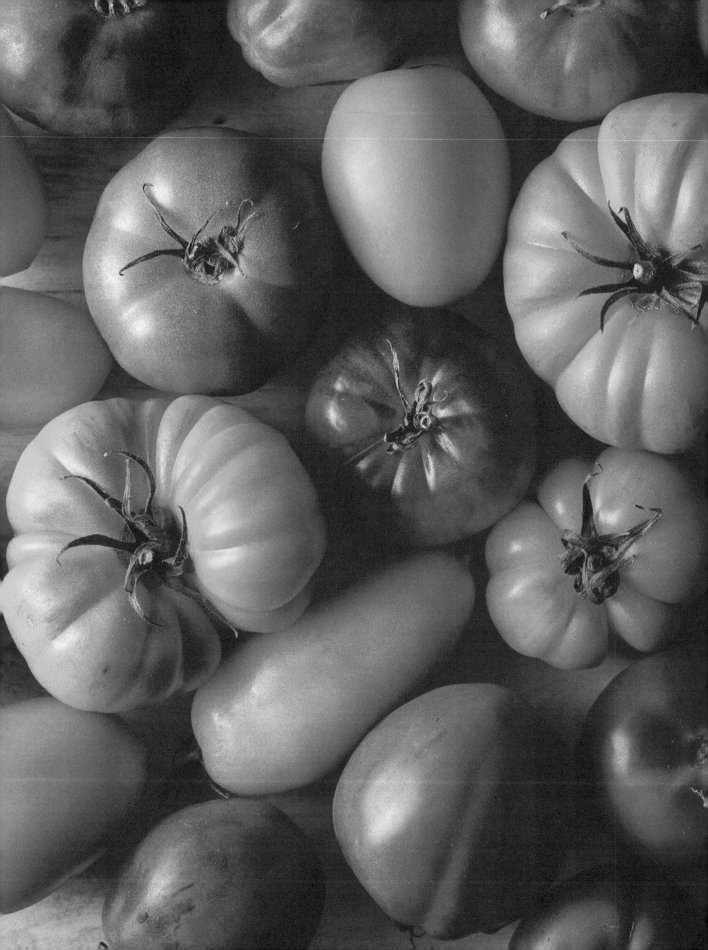

SOUPS AND SALADS

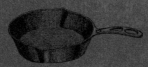

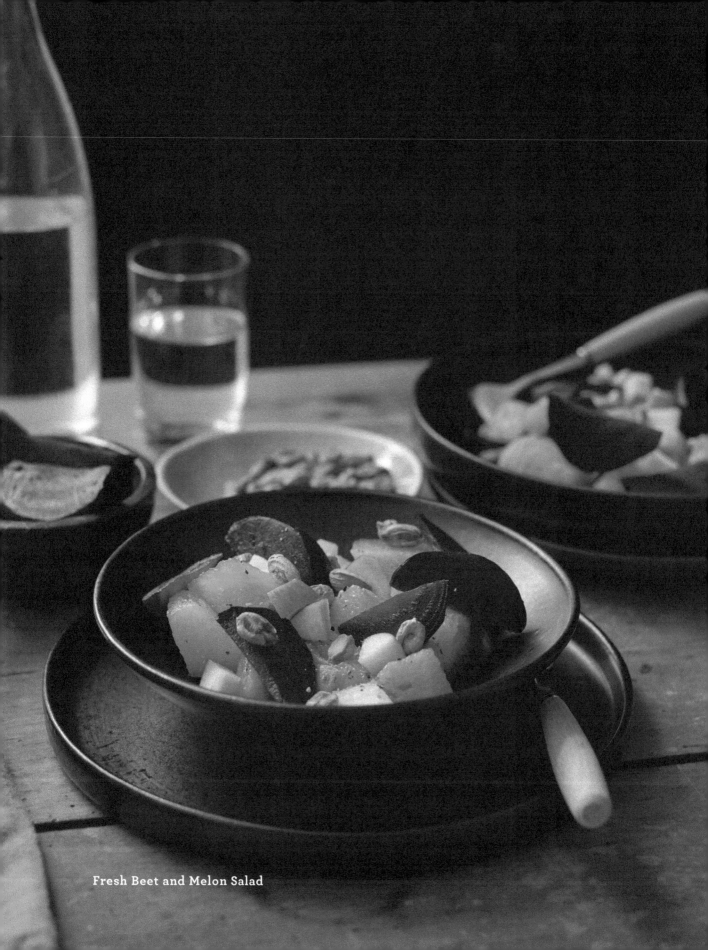

Fresh Beet and Melon Salad

FRESH BEET AND MELON SALAD

SERVES 4 | PREP TIME: **10 MINUTES** | COOK TIME: **30 MINUTES**

Mix a bit of summer and a bit of fall with this fresh salad. Enjoy the sweetness of the beets and watermelon with the crunch of pistachios in every bite.

2 medium beets, peeled

2 cups watermelon, cut into 1-inch chunks

1 cup chopped apples

¼ cup shelled pistachios

Juice of 1 lemon

1 teaspoon sea salt

1 teaspoon freshly ground black pepper

1. Preheat the oven to 400°F.

2. Tightly wrap the beets individually in aluminum foil and bake for 30 minutes or until fork-tender. Set aside to cool.

3. In a large bowl, combine the watermelon, apples, pistachios, lemon juice, salt, and pepper.

4. Cut the beets into ½-inch pieces and add to the watermelon mixture. Stir to combine and serve.

> Variation Tip: If you can handle small amounts of dairy, crumble ¼ cup of goat cheese over the salad.

PER SERVING CALORIES: 132; TOTAL FAT: 4G; SATURATED FAT: 1G; PROTEIN: 3G; TOTAL CARBOHYDRATES: 21G; FIBER: 4G; CHOLESTEROL: 0MG; MACROS: FAT: 27%; PROTEIN: 9%; CARBS: 64%

STRABERRY-WALNUT SUMMER SALAD

EASY, EGG-FREE, QUICK PREP, UNDER 30 MINUTES

SERVES 1 | PREP TIME: 10 MINUTES

This quick and easy salad highlights the rich and savory flavors of the walnuts and bacon.

2 cups baby spinach leaves

3 strawberries, cut into ¼-inch-thick slices

¼ cup roughly chopped walnuts

3 tablespoons finely chopped red onion

2 tablespoons nitrate- and sugar-free bacon slices, cooked and crumbled

Strawberry Balsamic Vinaigrette (page 230)

1. Arrange the spinach on a plate.

2. Top with the strawberries, walnuts, onion, and bacon.

3. Dress with the vinaigrette and serve.

Variation Tip: Walnuts can be swapped out for an equal amount of almonds, pistachios, or pecans.

PER SERVING CALORIES: 430; TOTAL FAT: 30G; SATURATED FAT: 5G; PROTEIN: 14G; TOTAL CARBOHYDRATES: 26G; FIBER: 5G; CHOLESTEROL: 21MG; MACROS: FAT: 63%; PROTEIN: 13%; CARBS: 24%

FRESH MINTED FRUIT SALAD

AIP-FRIENDLY, ALLERGEN-FREE, EASY, EGG-FREE, NUT-FREE, QUICK PREP, UNDER 30 MINUTES

SERVES 6 TO 8 | PREP TIME: 15 MINUTES, PLUS 30 MINUTES TO CHILL

Refresh your palate with the sweetness of stone fruit and the bold flavor of mint in each bite.

1 pound cherries, pitted and chopped

1 pound peaches, pitted and chopped

1 pound mango, chopped

1 pound nectarines, chopped

¼ cup freshly squeezed orange juice

1 tablespoon raw honey

¼ cup chopped fresh mint

1. In a large bowl, combine the cherries, peaches, mango, and nectarines.

2. In a small bowl, whisk together the orange juice and honey and fold in the mint.

3. Pour the dressing over the fruit salad and stir to fully coat. Serve cold.

> **Variation Tip:** Switch up this fruit-forward recipe by adding bananas, blueberries, or strawberries.

PER SERVING (½ CUP) CALORIES: 129; TOTAL FAT: 1G; SATURATED FAT: 0G; PROTEIN: 2G; TOTAL CARBOHYDRATES: 28G; FIBER: 4G; CHOLESTEROL: 0MG; MACROS: FAT: 7%; PROTEIN: 6%; CARBS: 87%

BROCCOLI, ALMOND, AND POPPY SEED SALAD

SERVES 4 | PREP TIME: 15 MINUTES

Each bite of this fresh salad is packed full of crunchy broccoli and almonds and sweetened to perfection with a deliciously addicting poppy seed dressing.

3 cups chopped
broccoli florets

⅓ cup slivered almonds

¼ cup finely chopped
red onion

4 nitrate- and sugar-free
bacon slices, cooked
and crumbled

¼ cup freshly squeezed
lemon juice

¼ cup extra-virgin olive oil

3 tablespoons raw honey

1 teaspoon spicy
brown mustard

1 teaspoon poppy seeds

¼ teaspoon sea salt

1. In a large bowl, combine the broccoli, almonds, onion, and bacon.

2. In a small bowl, whisk together the lemon juice, olive oil, honey, mustard, poppy seeds, and salt. Pour the dressing over the salad, stir to fully coat, and serve.

> Variation Tip: Swap out honey for pure maple syrup.

PER SERVING CALORIES: 353; TOTAL FAT: 25G; SATURATED FAT: 5G; PROTEIN: 11G; TOTAL CARBOHYDRATES: 21G; FIBER: 3G; CHOLESTEROL: 21MG; MACROS: FAT: 64%; PROTEIN: 12%; CARBS: 24%

GRILLED BUFFALO CHICKEN SALAD

EASY, NUT-FREE, QUICK PREP

SERVES 2 | PREP TIME: **15 MINUTES** | COOK TIME: **15 MINUTES**

Any true fan of buffalo wings will appreciate the classic buffalo chicken flavor throughout this vibrant and spicy salad.

1 tablespoon extra-virgin
   olive oil

2 (8-ounce) chicken breasts

Sea salt

Freshly ground black pepper

½ cup paleo-approved hot
   sauce, divided

1 tablespoon ghee

1 head romaine lettuce,
   roughly chopped

½ medium red onion, cut
   into ¼-inch-thick slices

1 medium avocado, sliced

1 medium celery stalk, cut
   into ¼-inch-thick slices

1 hard-boiled egg, chopped

6 nitrate- and sugar-free
   bacon slices, cooked
   and crumbled

Creamy Ranch Dressing
   (page 236), for serving

1. Heat the olive oil in a cast iron skillet over medium-high heat or preheat a grill to medium heat (about 375°F). Brush both sides of each chicken breast with the olive oil.

2. Season the chicken with the salt and pepper.

3. Cook the chicken breasts for 6 minutes (over indirect heat, if grilling), flip, and cook for an additional 6 minutes (or until deep grill marks appear, if grilling).

4. Using ¼ cup of the hot sauce, brush both sides of the chicken generously and grill for an additional 2 minutes or until the juices run clear and the internal temperature reaches 165°F. Remove from the heat and set aside.

5. In a small saucepan, combine the remaining ¼ cup of hot sauce and the ghee ⬛⬛⬛⬛ at for 3 minutes or until the ghee melts c⬛⬛⬛⬛ove from the heat.

6. Slice the chicken and c⬛⬛⬛⬛auce mixture.

7. Assemble the salad with th⬛⬛⬛⬛, onion, avocado, celery, egg, and bacon. Top with the buffalo chicken and homemade ranch dressing before serving.

> Ingredient Tip: Because the avocado will oxidize and turn brown, this salad is best eaten right away.

PER SERVING CALORIES: 1,126; TOTAL FAT: 82G; SATURATED FAT: 16G; PROTEIN: 77G; TOTAL CARBOHYDRATES: 20G; FIBER: 8G; CHOLESTEROL: 167MG; MACROS: FAT: 66%; PROTEIN: 27%; CARBS: 7%

GARDEN-FRESH TOMATO AND BASIL SOUP

SERVES 4 TO 6 | PREP TIME: **10 MINUTES** | COOK TIME: **20 MINUTES**

There is nothing more comforting than a big bowl of garden-fresh tomato soup packed full of hearty and earthy flavors.

2 tablespoons avocado oil

1 medium white onion, cut into ¼-inch-thick slices

3 medium garlic cloves, minced

3 pounds Roma tomatoes, cored

4 cups Chicken Bone Broth (page 28)

1 (6-ounce) can tomato paste

½ cup full-fat coconut milk

1 teaspoon sea salt

½ teaspoon freshly ground black pepper

½ teaspoon garlic

⅓ cup finely cho
fresh basil

1. Heat the avocado oil in a large stockpot over medium-high heat for 3 minutes or until the oil starts to shimmer.

2. Sauté the onion and garlic for 3 minutes or until the onion is translucent.

3. Add the tomatoes and bone broth and bring to a boil.

4. Cover and boil for 10 minutes or until the tomatoes begin to soften.

5. Transfer the tomato soup to a food processor. Add the tomato paste, coconut milk, salt, pepper, and garlic powder. Blend on high for 1 minute or until smooth.

6. Fold in the basil and serve.

> **Variation Tip:** If you prefer to work with canned tomatoes, use 3 (28-ounce) cans of fire-roasted crushed tomatoes.

PER SERVING (1 CUP) CALORIES: 303; TOTAL FAT: 15G; SATURATED FAT: 7G; PROTEIN: 15G; TOTAL CARBOHYDRATES: 27G; FIBER: 7G; CHOLESTEROL: 0MG; MACROS: FAT: 45%; PROTEIN: 19%; CARBS: 36%

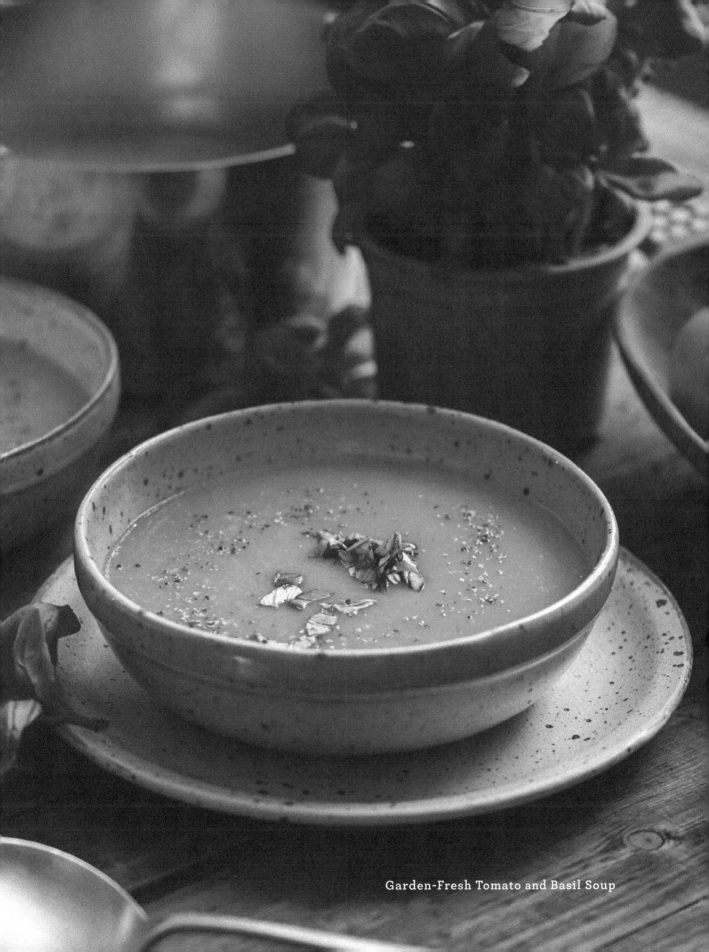

Garden-Fresh Tomato and Basil Soup

GRILLED MEXICAN-STYLE CHICKEN AND AVOCADO SALAD

EASY, NUT-FREE, QUICK PREP, UNDER 30 MINUTES

SERVES 2 | PREP TIME: **5 MINUTES** | COOK TIME: **15 MINUTES**

Savor creamy avocados, spicy taco seasoning, and fresh cilantro in every bite of this lively salad.

1 tablespoon extra-virgin olive oil

2 (8-ounce) chicken breasts

2 tablespoons Two-Minute Taco Seasoning (page 231)

2 medium avocados

¼ cup Real Paleo Mayonnaise (page 234)

1 tablespoon chopped fresh cilantro

2 teaspoons freshly squeezed lime juice

½ teaspoon sea salt

¼ cup finely chopped red onion

3 medium garlic cloves, minced

1. Heat the olive oil in a cast iron skillet over medium-high heat or preheat a grill to medium heat (about 375°F). Brush both sides of each chicken breast with olive oil.

2. Season the chicken with the taco seasoning.

3. Cook the chicken breasts for 6 minutes (over indirect heat, if grilling), flip, and cook for an additional 6 minutes (or until deep grill marks appear and the juices run clear, if grilling). The internal temperature should reach 165°F. Remove from the heat and set aside.

4. In a medium bowl, mash the avocados until smooth and creamy.

5. Fold in the mayonnaise, cilantro, lime juice, and salt.

6. Cut the chicken into ½-inch-thick slices and fold it, with the red onion and garlic, into the mashed avocados. Serve immediately.

> Storage Tip: This dish is best eaten right away, but if you must store it longer, put it into an airtight storage container in the refrigerator for up to 2 days. The longer the salad is kept, the more the avocado will oxidize and turn brown.

PER SERVING CALORIES: 943; TOTAL FAT: 71G; SATURATED FAT: 9G; PROTEIN: 56G; TOTAL CARBOHYDRATES: 20G; FIBER: 12G; CHOLESTEROL: 24MG; MACROS: FAT: 68%; PROTEIN: 24%; CARBS: 8%

CREAMY MUSHROOM SOUP

AIP-FRIENDLY, ALLERGEN-FREE, EASY, EGG-FREE, QUICK PREP, UNDER 30 MINUTES

SERVES 4 | PREP TIME: 10 MINUTES | COOK TIME: 10 MINUTES

This creamy, dairy-free soup will take you back to your childhood with its comforting mushroom flavor.

1½ cups Chicken Bone Broth (page 28)

5 cups cremini or baby bella mushrooms, cut into ¼-inch-thick slices

½ cup chopped white onion

⅛ teaspoon dried thyme

3 tablespoons coconut oil

3 tablespoons arrowroot flour

1 cup coconut cream

½ teaspoon onion powder

¼ teaspoon sea salt

½ teaspoon freshly ground black pepper

1. Heat the bone broth, mushrooms, onion, and thyme in a large stockpot over medium-high heat and bring to a boil.

2. Cover, reduce the heat to low, and simmer for 10 minutes or until the mushrooms are fork-tender.

3. Transfer to a food processor and blend on high for 30 seconds or until smooth. Set aside.

4. Return the stockpot to the burner and heat the coconut oil over medium-high heat for 2 minutes or until completely melted.

5. Whisk in the arrowroot flour for 30 seconds or until thick and smooth.

6. Add the mushroom mixture, coconut cream, onion powder, salt, and pepper. Stir for 1 minute or until thickened. Serve.

Ingredient Tip: If you don't have coconut cream on hand, use the fat from a can of coconut milk.

PER SERVING CALORIES: 315; TOTAL FAT: 23G; SATURATED FAT: 20G; PROTEIN: 17G; TOTAL CARBOHYDRATES: 10G; FIBER: 2G; CHOLESTEROL: 0MG; MACROS: FAT: 66%; PROTEIN: 22%; CARBS: 12%

CREAMY CAULIFLOWER SOUP

AIP-FRIENDLY, ALLERGEN-FREE, EASY, EGG-FREE, QUICK PREP

SERVES 4 TO 6 | PREP TIME: **10 MINUTES** | COOK TIME: **25 MINUTES**

This soup is packed full of creamy cauliflower with hints of chive and bacon bits throughout.

6 nitrate- and sugar-free bacon slices, chopped

½ medium white onion, chopped

3 medium garlic cloves, minced

1 (13.5-ounce) can full-fat coconut milk

3 cups Chicken Bone Broth (page 28)

1 large head cauliflower, chopped

1 teaspoon sea salt

½ teaspoon freshly ground black pepper

Chopped fresh chives, for garnish

1. Cook the bacon in a large stockpot over medium-high heat for 5 minutes or until brown and crispy.

2. With a slotted spoon, transfer the bacon to a paper towel–lined plate to remove the excess grease. Set aside.

3. In the pot with the bacon grease, add the onion and garlic and cook for 3 minutes or until the onion is translucent.

4. Add the coconut milk, bone broth, cauliflower, salt, and pepper and bring to a boil.

5. Cover, reduce the heat to low, and simmer for 15 minutes or until the cauliflower is fork-tender.

6. Transfer the cauliflower soup to a food processor and blend on high for 2 minutes or until smooth and creamy.

7. Add additional salt and pepper to taste. Serve topped with chives and the bacon.

> **Variation Tip:** Coconut milk can be swapped out for almond milk.

PER SERVING (1 CUP) CALORIES: 487; TOTAL FAT: 35G; SATURATED FAT: 24G; PROTEIN: 24G; TOTAL CARBOHYDRATES: 19G; FIBER: 8G; CHOLESTEROL: 31MG; MACROS: FAT: 65%; PROTEIN: 19%; CARBS: 16%

SEAFOOD BISQUE

EASY, EGG-FREE, QUICK PREP, UNDER 30 MINUTES

SERVES 4 | PREP TIME: **10 MINUTES** | COOK TIME: **15 MINUTES**

This dish is super simple and flavorful. Packed with seafood and vegetables, this bisque will satisfy any seafood craving.

2 tablespoons avocado oil

2 tablespoons finely chopped scallions, white and green parts

2 tablespoons finely chopped celery

3 tablespoons arrowroot flour

3 cups full-fat coconut milk

1 tablespoon tomato paste

1 cup coconut cream

2 tablespoons sherry

½ teaspoon freshly ground black pepper

8 ounces shredded crab meat

8 ounces cooked shrimp, chopped

1. Heat the avocado oil in a large stockpot over medium-high heat for 3 minutes or until the oil starts to shimmer.

2. Sauté the scallions and celery for 3 minutes or until fork-tender.

3. Whisk in the arrowroot flour for 30 seconds or until a smooth white paste forms.

4. Slowly add the coconut milk while whisking for 1 minute or until thickened.

5. Add the tomato paste, coconut cream, sherry, and pepper, then fold in the crab meat and shrimp.

6. Cover, reduce the heat to low, and simmer for 10 minutes or until the crab meat is white and tender. Serve immediately.

> Variation Tip: Swap out the crab and shrimp for lobster, scallops, or any flaky white fish to make this your own unique and flavorful dish.

PER SERVING CALORIES: 756; TOTAL FAT: 64G; SATURATED FAT: 51G; PROTEIN: 26G; TOTAL CARBOHYDRATES: 19G; FIBER: 5G; CHOLESTEROL: 150MG; MACROS: FAT: 76%; PROTEIN: 14%; CARBS: 10%

CLASSIC CHICKEN SOUP

AIP-FRIENDLY, ALLERGEN-FREE, EASY, EGG-FREE, NUT-FREE, QUICK PREP

SERVES 4 | PREP TIME: **10 MINUTES** | COOK TIME: **30 MINUTES**

Enjoy a warm bowl of this classic and comforting chicken soup loaded with sweet vegetables and a savory hint of fresh parsley.

¼ cup extra-virgin olive oil

1 medium white
   onion, diced

3 medium carrots, cut into
   ¼-inch-thick slices

4 medium celery stalks,
   finely chopped

3 medium garlic
   cloves, minced

1 teaspoon sea salt

1 teaspoon freshly ground
   black pepper

8 cups Chicken Bone Broth
   (page 28)

4 cups cooked and
   shredded chicken breast

½ cup chopped
   fresh parsley

1. Heat the olive oil in a large stockpot over medium heat for 3 minutes or until the oil starts to shimmer.

2. Sauté the onion, carrots, celery, and garlic with the salt and pepper for 5 minutes or until the vegetables are soft and fragrant.

3. Add the bone broth and bring to a gentle boil.

4. Cover, reduce the heat to low, and simmer for 15 minutes.

5. Add the chicken and parsley and season with additional salt and pepper as desired, then serve.

Variation Tip: Make a chicken and "rice" soup by adding Grated Cauliflower Rice (page 37) during step 3.

PER SERVING CALORIES: 497; TOTAL FAT: 24G; SATURATED FAT: 5G; PROTEIN: 61G; TOTAL CARBOHYDRATES: 10G; FIBER: 3G; CHOLESTEROL: 118MG; MACROS: FAT: 43%; PROTEIN: 49%; CARBS: 8%

SOUTHWEST CHILI

ALLERGEN-FREE, EASY, EGG-FREE, NUT-FREE, QUICK PREP

SERVES 4 | PREP TIME: 10 MINUTES | COOK TIME: 30 MINUTES

This chili will become a family favorite with its Southwestern-style spicy kick. Make this dish for your next game night, or warm up with a bowl tonight!

1 pound 80/20 ground beef

½ medium white onion, diced

1 (14-ounce) can tomato sauce

1 (14-ounce) can diced tomatoes with green chiles

1 tablespoon chili powder

1 tablespoon ground cumin

1 teaspoon ground paprika

1 teaspoon garlic powder

½ teaspoon sea salt

¼ teaspoon freshly ground black pepper

1. Heat the ground beef and onion in a large skillet over medium-high heat for 5 minutes or until browned and no longer visibly pink.

2. Add the tomato sauce, diced tomatoes with their juices, chili powder, cumin, paprika, garlic powder, salt, and pepper. Bring to a gentle boil.

3. Cover, reduce the heat to low, and cook for an additional 20 minutes or until thick and fragrant. Serve immediately.

Variation Tip: For a lighter chili, use turkey or chicken instead of ground beef.

PER SERVING CALORIES: 328; TOTAL FAT: 20G; SATURATED FAT: 8G; PROTEIN: 24G; TOTAL CARBOHYDRATES: 13G; FIBER: 3G; CHOLESTEROL: 59MG; MACROS: FAT: 55%; PROTEIN: 29%; CARBS: 16%

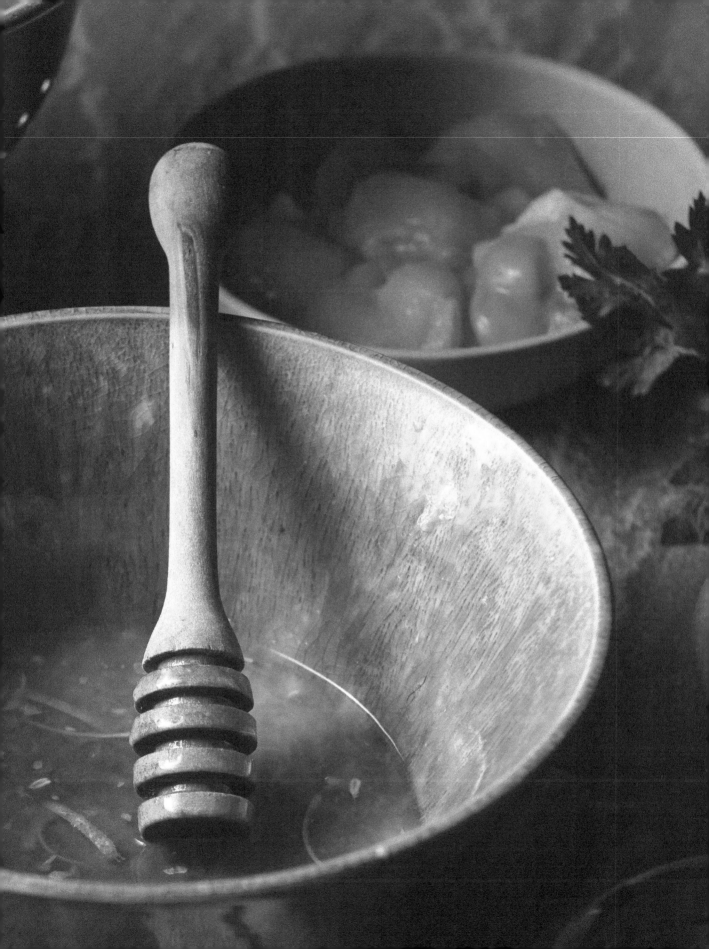

CHAPTER EIGHT

FISH AND SEAFOOD

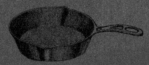

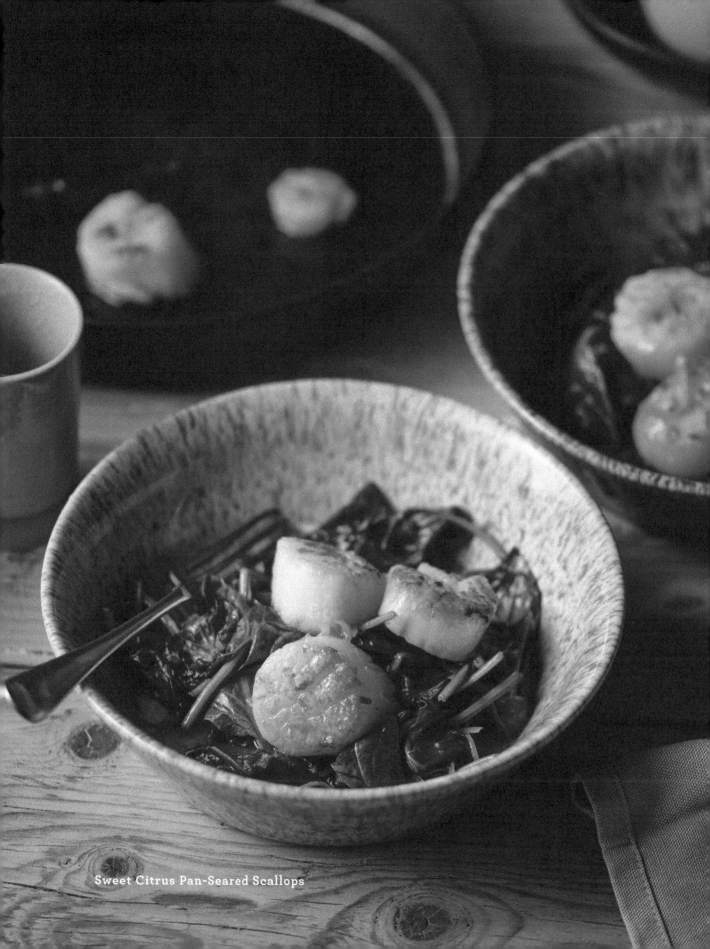

Sweet Citrus Pan-Seared Scallops

SWEET CITRUS PAN-SEARED SCALLOPS

AIP-FRIENDLY, EGG-FREE, NUT-FREE, QUICK PREP, UNDER 30 MINUTES

SERVES 4 | PREP TIME: **10 MINUTES** | COOK TIME: **5 MINUTES**

These simple yet beautiful pan-seared scallops are restaurant quality. Enjoy them topped with a sweet, honey-kissed citrus dressing.

FOR THE SCALLOPS

1 pound large sea scallops

2 tablespoons avocado oil

Sea salt

Freshly ground black pepper

FOR THE CITRUS DRESSING

2 tablespoons freshly squeezed lemon juice

1 tablespoon raw honey

¼ teaspoon sea salt

TO MAKE THE SCALLOPS

1. Rinse the scallops and place them on a paper towel. Cover with a second paper towel and gently pat to soak up excess moisture. Leave covered for 10 minutes.

2. Heat the avocado oil in a cast iron skillet over medium-high heat for 10 minutes or until the oil starts to shimmer.

3. Season both sides of the scallops generously with salt and pepper.

4. Sear the scallops for 2 minutes, flip, and cook for an additional 1½ to 2 minutes or until they are opaque and slightly browned. Transfer the scallops to a plate and cover loosely with aluminum foil.

TO MAKE THE CITRUS DRESSING

1. In a small bowl, whisk together the lemon juice, honey, and salt.

2. Drizzle the sauce over the pan-seared scallops and serve.

> Ingredient Tip: Serve the scallops over a bed of lettuce, or pair them with a side of sautéed greens such as spinach, chard, or kale.

PER SERVING CALORIES: 176; TOTAL FAT: 8G; SATURATED FAT: 1G; PROTEIN: 19G; TOTAL CARBOHYDRATES: 7G; FIBER: 0G; CHOLESTEROL: 37MG; MACROS: FAT: 41%; PROTEIN: 43%; CARBS: 16%

GRILLED SHRIMP AND PINEAPPLE SKEWERS

EASY, EGG-FREE, NUT-FREE, QUICK PREP

SERVES 4 | PREP TIME: 10 MINUTES, PLUS 20 MINUTES TO MARINATE | COOK TIME: **10 MINUTES**

These grilled shrimp and pineapple skewers make a fun appetizer or a low-carbohydrate meal any day of the week.

---

12 raw jumbo shrimp, washed, peeled, and deveined

1 medium red onion, quartered

½ pineapple, cut into 2-inch chunks

1 tablespoon extra-virgin olive oil

1 garlic clove, minced

1 teaspoon chopped shallot

1 teaspoon freshly squeezed lemon juice

½ teaspoon ground coriander

¼ teaspoon red pepper flakes

¼ teaspoon sea salt

1. Preheat a cast iron pan over medium-high heat or a grill to medium heat (about 375°F). If using wooden skewers, start soaking them in water.

2. In a large bowl, combine the shrimp, onion, pineapple, olive oil, garlic, shallot, lemon juice, coriander, red pepper flakes, and salt.

3. Set the shrimp mixture in the refrigerator for 20 minutes to marinate.

4. Thread the skewers by alternating shrimp, pineapple, and onion until all the ingredients are used.

5. Put the threaded skewers onto the preheated grill or in the cast iron pan and cook for 3 minutes. Flip the skewers and cook for an additional 3 minutes until the shrimp is pink and firm. Serve immediately.

> **Prep Tip:** Marinate the shrimp, red onion, and pineapple overnight for faster meal prep.

PER SERVING CALORIES: 147; TOTAL FAT: 4G; SATURATED FAT: 1G; PROTEIN: 13G; TOTAL CARBOHYDRATES: 14G; FIBER: 2G; CHOLESTEROL: 111MG; MACROS: FAT: 24%; PROTEIN: 35%; CARBS: 41%

PERFECTLY MARINATED SALMON

AIP-FRIENDLY, EASY, EGG-FREE, QUICK PREP

SERVES 2 | PREP TIME: 10 MINUTES, PLUS 10 MINUTES TO MARINATE | COOK TIME: 15 MINUTES

Enjoy the sweet hints of honey and coconut aminos and the savory hints of garlic and parsley in this salmon dish.

---

2 (4-ounce) fresh wild-caught salmon fillets

4 tablespoons extra-virgin olive oil

1 tablespoon coconut aminos

1 tablespoon raw honey

2 teaspoons finely chopped fresh parsley

1 garlic clove, minced

1 teaspoon freshly squeezed lemon juice

½ teaspoon freshly ground black pepper

¼ teaspoon sea salt

1. Preheat the oven to 425°F. Line an edged baking sheet with parchment paper.

2. In a resealable quart-size bag, combine the salmon fillets, olive oil, coconut aminos, honey, parsley, garlic, lemon juice, pepper, and salt. Marinate the salmon unrefrigerated for 10 minutes.

3. Remove the salmon and place it on the prepared baking sheet. Bake for 15 minutes or until the salmon has a slightly translucent pink center with an internal temperature of 145°F.

4. Let the salmon rest for 5 minutes before serving.

> Ingredient Tip: Marinate the salmon in the refrigerator for 4 to 6 hours for a more intense flavor.

PER SERVING CALORIES: 449; TOTAL FAT: 33G; SATURATED FAT: 5G; PROTEIN: 27G; TOTAL CARBOHYDRATES: 11G; FIBER: 0G; CHOLESTEROL: 60MG; MACROS: FAT: 66%; PROTEIN: 24%; CARBS: 10%

BAKED CHIMICHURRI HALIBUT

EASY, EGG-FREE, NUT-FREE, QUICK PREP, UNDER 30 MINUTES

SERVES 2 | PREP TIME: **10 MINUTES** | COOK TIME: **15 MINUTES**

Elevate your baked halibut with this traditional Argentinian-inspired chimichurri sauce, a versatile and fantastic addition to fish, beef, and chicken.

FOR THE HALIBUT

2 (6-ounce) halibut fillets

1 tablespoon extra-virgin olive oil

Sea salt

Freshly ground black pepper

FOR THE CHIMICHURRI SAUCE

½ cup extra-virgin olive oil

¼ cup chopped fresh parsley

4 medium garlic cloves, minced

2 tablespoons red wine vinegar

2 tablespoons dried oregano

2 teaspoons red pepper flakes

TO MAKE THE HALIBUT

1. Preheat the oven to 400°F. Line an edged baking sheet with parchment paper.

2. Place the halibut fillets on the prepared baking sheet and brush with the olive oil.

3. Season the fish with the salt and pepper.

4. Bake for 15 minutes or until the halibut is flaky.

TO MAKE THE CHIMICHURRI SAUCE

1. In a food processor, add the olive oil, parsley, garlic, vinegar, oregano, and red pepper flakes. Pulse 20 to 30 times or until the sauce is smooth yet still slightly chunky.

2. Spread the sauce over the halibut fillets and serve.

Variation Tip: For an AIP-friendly dish, omit the chimichurri. Instead, squeeze fresh lemon juice onto the fillets and enjoy.

PER SERVING CALORIES: 711; TOTAL FAT: 55G; SATURATED FAT: 7G; PROTEIN: 47G; TOTAL CARBOHYDRATES: 7G; FIBER: 3G; CHOLESTEROL: 79MG; MACROS: FAT: 70%; PROTEIN: 26%; CARBS: 4%

SHRIMP SCAMPI

EGG-FREE, NUT-FREE, QUICK PREP

SERVES 4 | PREP TIME: 10 MINUTES | COOK TIME: 20 MINUTES

Turn your traditional shrimp scampi into a flavor-packed meal tossed with zucchini noodles.

2 tablespoons ghee, divided

1 pound small shrimp, washed, peeled, and deveined

5 large garlic cloves, minced

2 shallots, chopped

¾ cup white wine

Juice of 1 lemon

½ teaspoon sea salt, plus more for seasoning

¼ teaspoon freshly ground black pepper, plus more for seasoning

¼ teaspoon red pepper flakes

¼ cup chopped fresh parsley

Zest of 1 lemon

Zucchini Noodles (Zoodles, page 32)

1 to 2 tablespoons extra-virgin olive oil

1. Heat 1 tablespoon of ghee in a large skillet over medium-high heat for 3 minutes or until melted and shimmering.

2. Pat the shrimp dry and season with salt and pepper.

3. Fry the shrimp in a single layer for 1 minute, then flip and cook for an additional minute. Remove from the skillet and set aside.

4. Return the skillet to the burner and sauté the garlic and shallots in the remaining 1 tablespoon of ghee over medium-high heat for 3 minutes or until soft and fragrant.

5. Add the white wine, lemon juice, salt, pepper, and red pepper flakes and deglaze the skillet, scraping and stirring up the browned bits from the bottom. Bring to a boil.

6. Boil for 5 minutes or until the liquid is reduced by half.

7. Turn the burner off and fold in the parsley, lemon zest, shrimp, and zoodles.

8. Cover for 5 minutes or until the shrimp are pink.

9. Toss with the olive oil and serve immediately.

Make-Ahead Tip: Make Zucchini Noodles (Zoodles, page 32) ahead—or use leftovers.

PER SERVING CALORIES: 263; TOTAL FAT: 15G; SATURATED FAT: 5G; PROTEIN: 25G; TOTAL CARBOHYDRATES: 7G; FIBER: 1G; CHOLESTEROL: 236MG; MACROS: FAT: 51%; PROTEIN: 38%; CARBS: 11%

FRIED COD DINNER

EASY, EGG-FREE, QUICK PREP, UNDER 30 MINUTES

SERVES 4 | PREP TIME: 10 MINUTES | COOK TIME: **10 MINUTES**

Bring the fish fry tradition home and make this delicious, mouthwatering fried fish in the comforts of your kitchen.

1 cup coconut oil

½ cup tapioca flour

⅓ cup unsweetened shredded coconut

1 teaspoon ground paprika

¼ teaspoon sea salt

½ teaspoon freshly ground black pepper

4 (6-ounce) cod fillets

1. Heat the coconut oil in a cast iron skillet over medium-high heat for 10 minutes or until the oil starts to shimmer.

2. In a medium bowl, combine the tapioca flour, coconut, paprika, salt, and pepper.

3. Dredge the cod fillets one at a time in the flour mixture, coating both sides generously.

4. Fry the fillets for 3 minutes, then flip and cook for an additional 3 minutes until they're brown and crisp. (Cod is cooked when the internal temperature reaches 145°F.)

5. Remove the fish from the skillet and place on a paper towel–lined plate to remove excess oil before serving.

Make-Ahead Tip: Make tartar sauce ahead of time by whisking together ½ cup of Real Paleo Mayonnaise (page 234), 3 tablespoons of finely chopped dill pickles, 1 tablespoon of lemon juice, 1 tablespoon of dill, 1 teaspoon of minced garlic, 1 teaspoon of stone-ground mustard, and ½ teaspoon of onion powder.

PER SERVING CALORIES: 377; TOTAL FAT: 21G; SATURATED FAT: 17G; PROTEIN: 31G; TOTAL CARBOHYDRATES: 16G; FIBER: 2G; CHOLESTEROL: 83MG; MACROS: FAT: 50%; PROTEIN: 33%; CARBS: 17%

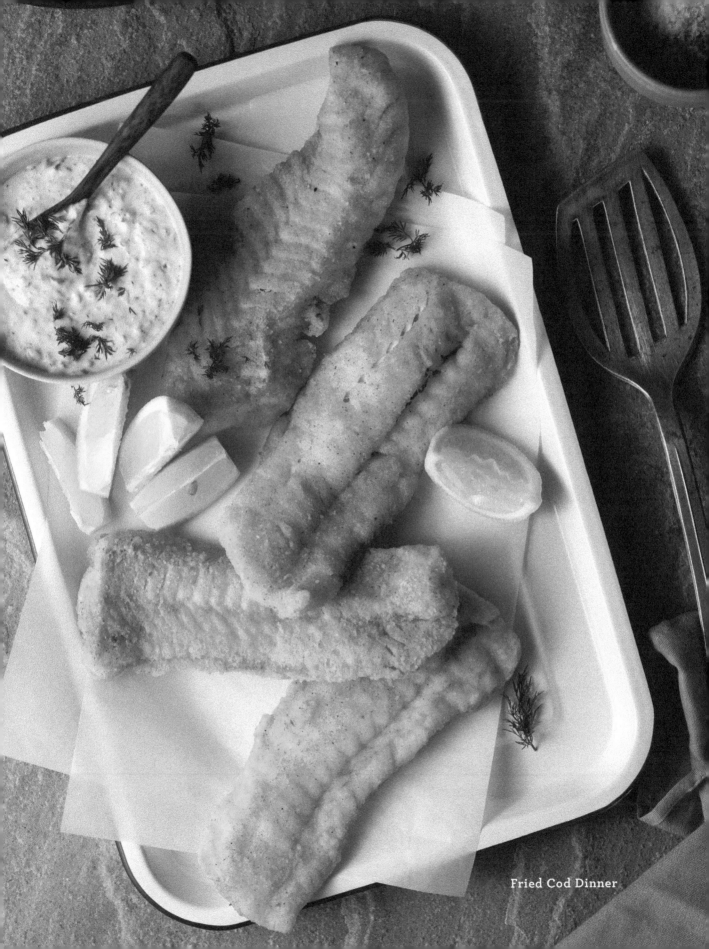

Fried Cod Dinner

BANG-BANG SHRIMP TACOS

EASY, QUICK PREP, UNDER 30 MINUTES

SERVES 4 | PREP TIME: **10 MINUTES** | COOK TIME: **10 MINUTES**

Get a bang in every bite with these bang-bang shrimp tacos!

2 tablespoons coconut oil

⅓ cup coconut flour

¼ cup arrowroot flour

1 teaspoon sea salt

1 large egg

1 pound small shrimp, peeled and deveined

¼ cup Real Paleo Mayonnaise (page 234)

2 tablespoons Sugar-Free Ketchup (page 235)

2 teaspoons coconut aminos

2 teaspoons paleo-approved hot sauce

1 garlic clove, minced

4 AIP/Allergen-Free Tortillas (page 36)

4 cups shredded lettuce

1. Heat the coconut oil in a large skillet over medium-high heat for 3 minutes or until the oil starts to shimmer.

2. In a small bowl, combine the coconut flour, arrowroot flour, and salt.

3. In another small bowl, whisk the egg. Dip the shrimp in the whisked egg and then dredge in the flour mixture, coating each side of the shrimp generously. Shake off any excess flour.

4. Fry the shrimp in a single layer for 4 minutes, then flip and cook for an additional 3 to 5 minutes or until the shrimp are golden brown and crispy. Transfer the shrimp to a large bowl.

5. In a small bowl, whisk together the mayonnaise, ketchup, coconut aminos, hot sauce, and garlic. Add the sauce to the shrimp and toss until evenly coated.

6. Divide the shrimp evenly among the tortillas, top with the lettuce, wrap, and serve immediately.

Make-Ahead Tip: Make the AIP/Allergen-Free Tortillas (page 36), Real Paleo Mayonnaise (page 234), and Sugar-Free Ketchup (page 235) ahead to save time.

PER SERVING CALORIES: 490; TOTAL FAT: 26G; SATURATED FAT: 12G; PROTEIN: 33G; TOTAL CARBOHYDRATES: 31G; FIBER: 13G; CHOLESTEROL: 299MG; MACROS: FAT: 48%; PROTEIN: 27%; CARBS: 25%

BAKED SALMON PATTIES

EASY, QUICK PREP, UNDER 30 MINUTES

SERVES 8 | PREP TIME: **10 MINUTES** | COOK TIME: **10 MINUTES**

Enjoy these rich salmon cakes as your main meal or as an appetizer with a side of spicy aioli for dipping.

3 (6-ounce) cans
   salmon, drained

1 large egg

1 scallion, white and green
   parts, chopped

1 tablespoon coconut flour

1 tablespoon
   stone-ground mustard

½ teaspoon sea salt

½ teaspoon freshly ground
   black pepper

1. Preheat the oven to 400°F. Line a baking sheet with parchment paper.

2. In a large bowl, combine the salmon, egg, scallion, coconut flour, mustard, salt, and pepper.

3. Divide the mixture into 8 equal balls. Flatten each ball between two pieces of parchment (or with your hands) to form ½-inch-thick patties.

4. Place the salmon patties on the prepared baking sheet and bake for 5 minutes, then flip and bake for an additional 5 minutes or until golden brown. Serve immediately.

Make-Ahead Tip: Make an accompanying homemade spicy aioli by whisking together ⅓ cup of Real Paleo Mayonnaise (page 234), ½ teaspoon of cayenne powder, and 2 minced garlic cloves.

PER SERVING CALORIES: 119; TOTAL FAT: 6G; SATURATED FAT: 1G; PROTEIN: 14G; TOTAL CARBOHYDRATES: 2G; FIBER: 1G; CHOLESTEROL: 51MG; MACROS: FAT: 45%; PROTEIN: 47%; CARBS: 8%

CREOLE SEAFOOD JAMBALAYA

SERVES 4 | PREP TIME: **10 MINUTES** | COOK TIME: **30 MINUTES**

Bring classic Creole flavors home with this zingy and vibrant seafood jambalaya.

2 tablespoons avocado oil

1 medium white
   onion, chopped

½ cup chopped celery

¼ cup chopped bell pepper

2 large garlic
   cloves, minced

1 (28-ounce) can
   diced tomatoes

1 cup Beef Bone Broth
   (page 27) or
   seafood broth

4 cups Grated Cauliflower
   Rice (page 37)

1 teaspoon sea salt

1 teaspoon garlic powder

1 teaspoon freshly ground
   black pepper

1 teaspoon dried thyme

1 teaspoon dried basil

1 teaspoon dried oregano

1 teaspoon ground paprika

1 teaspoon onion powder

½ teaspoon cayenne powder

8 ounces bay scallops

8 ounces shrimp, peeled
   and deveined

8 ounces shredded
   crab meat

1. Heat the avocado oil in a Dutch oven or stockpot over medium-high heat for 3 minutes or until the oil starts to shimmer.

2. Sauté the onion, celery, bell pepper, and garlic for 3 minutes or until the vegetables are fragrant and soft.

3. Add the tomatoes, bone broth, cauliflower rice, salt, garlic powder, pepper, thyme, basil, oregano, paprika, onion powder, and cayenne. Bring to a boil.

4. Cover, reduce the heat to low, and simmer for 15 minutes or until the cauliflower rice is tender.

5. Add the scallops, shrimp, and crab meat and simmer uncovered for 10 minutes or until the shrimp are pink and opaque and the scallops and crab meat are white and cooked thoroughly. Serve immediately.

Variation Tip: Scallops, shrimp, and crab meat aren't the only options for this zippy stew. Substitute or add your favorite seafood to make your own rendition of this dish.

PER SERVING CALORIES: 295; TOTAL FAT: 9G; SATURATED FAT: 1G; PROTEIN: 33G; TOTAL CARBOHYDRATES: 21G; FIBER: 6G; CHOLESTEROL: 109MG; MACROS: FAT: 27%; PROTEIN: 45%; CARBS: 28%

SEAFOOD STEW

EASY, EGG-FREE, NUT-FREE, ONE-POT, QUICK PREP

SERVES 4 | PREP TIME: 10 MINUTES | COOK TIME: 4 HOURS

Enjoy a seafood-packed stew with enticing flavors—subtle hints of red pepper and cayenne pepper along with earthy fresh seafood.

1 (28-ounce) can crushed tomatoes

4 cups Chicken Bone Broth (page 28)

3 medium garlic cloves, minced

½ cup chopped white onion

½ cup chopped carrots

½ cup chopped celery

1 teaspoon dried basil

1 teaspoon dried thyme

½ teaspoon sea salt

½ teaspoon freshly ground black pepper

½ teaspoon celery salt

¼ teaspoon red pepper flakes

⅛ teaspoon ground cayenne pepper

8 ounces frozen shrimp, peeled and deveined

1 pound frozen blue mussels

8 ounces frozen bay scallops

8 ounces frozen calamari

1. In a 6-quart or larger slow cooker, combine the tomatoes, bone broth, garlic, onion, carrots, celery, basil, thyme, salt, pepper, celery salt, red pepper flakes, and cayenne.

2. Cover and cook on low for 2 to 4 hours or until the carrots are fork-tender.

3. While the stew is cooking, put the frozen shrimp, mussels, scallops, and calamari into a resealable quart-size bag, seal, and immerse in a large bowl of cold water for 1 hour. Remove from the bowl and refrigerate while the vegetables cook.

4. When the vegetables are done, add the thawed shrimp, mussels, scallops, and calamari to the slow cooker and cook for an additional 1 hour on high or until the shrimp is pink and the scallops are opaque. Serve immediately.

Prep Tip: Place the frozen seafood in the refrigerator the night before to thaw overnight.

PER SERVING CALORIES: 323; TOTAL FAT: 3G; SATURATED FAT: 1G; PROTEIN: 55G; TOTAL CARBOHYDRATES: 19G; FIBER: 8G; CHOLESTEROL: 245MG; MACROS: FAT: 8%; PROTEIN: 68%; CARBS: 24%

CREAMY TUSCAN SALMON

SERVES 4 | PREP TIME: **10 MINUTES** | COOK TIME: **20 MINUTES**

Enjoy hints of garlic in this lush salmon dish mixed with sweet and tart sun-dried tomatoes and earthy spinach.

2 tablespoons avocado oil

4 (6-ounce) salmon fillets, skin removed

2 tablespoons ghee

6 medium garlic cloves, minced

1 medium white onion, chopped

¼ cup chopped sun-dried tomatoes

1½ cups full-fat coconut milk

½ teaspoon sea salt, plus more for seasoning

½ teaspoon freshly ground black pepper, plus more for seasoning

3 cups chopped baby spinach

1 tablespoon arrowroot flour

1 tablespoon warm water

1 tablespoon chopped fresh parsley

1. Heat the avocado oil in a large skillet over medium-high heat for 3 minutes or until the oil starts to shimmer.

2. Season the salmon fillets with salt and pepper.

3. Sear the salmon fillets for 5 minutes, then flip and cook for an additional 5 minutes or until the salmon has a slightly translucent pink center with an internal temperature of 145°F. Remove from the skillet and set aside.

4. Heat the ghee in the skillet over medium-high heat for 2 minutes or until melted.

5. Sauté the garlic and onion for 1 to 2 minutes or until fragrant. Add the sun-dried tomatoes and sauté for 1 minute or until softened.

6. Reduce the heat to low, whisk in the coconut milk, salt, and pepper. Bring to a simmer. Add the spinach, stirring until it is gently wilted.

7. In a small bowl, whisk together the arrowroot flour and warm water. Stir the mixture into the sauce for 30 seconds or until it starts to thicken.

8. Return the salmon to the sauce in the pan, sprinkle with the parsley, and serve.

> Variation Tip: Halibut and bass are equally good in this recipe and offer a lighter flavor.

PER SERVING CALORIES: 673; TOTAL FAT: 53G; SATURATED FAT: 28G; PROTEIN: 37G; TOTAL CARBOHYDRATES: 12G; FIBER: 4G; CHOLESTEROL: 114MG; MACROS: FAT: 71%; PROTEIN: 22%; CARBS: 7%

BLACKENED GROUPER WRAP

SERVES 4 | PREP TIME: **5 MINUTES** | COOK TIME: **10 MINUTES**

Sweet and savory flavors come through in every bite of this easily prepared, perfectly seasoned grouper wrap.

¾ teaspoon garlic powder

½ teaspoon sea salt

½ teaspoon freshly ground black pepper

1½ teaspoons ground paprika

1 teaspoon dried oregano

½ teaspoon ground cumin

1½ teaspoons coconut sugar

3 tablespoons avocado oil, divided

4 (6-ounce) grouper fillets

1 head butter lettuce

Real Paleo Mayonnaise (page 234)

1. In a small bowl, combine the garlic powder, salt, pepper, paprika, oregano, cumin, and coconut sugar. Set aside.

2. Heat 2 tablespoons of avocado oil in a cast iron skillet over medium-high heat for 5 minutes or until the oil starts to shimmer.

3. Brush both sides of the grouper fillets with the remaining 1 tablespoon of avocado oil, then coat them with the seasoning mix.

4. Cook the grouper fillets for 3 minutes, then flip and cook for an additional 3 minutes or until the fish is flaky and its internal temperature reaches 145°F.

5. Remove the fillets from the skillet. Place each fillet on a lettuce bed, add homemade mayonnaise, and roll it into a wrap. Serve immediately.

Storage Tip: Store leftover grouper fillets in the refrigerator in an airtight container separate from the lettuce and mayonnaise. Best if eaten within 2 days.

PER SERVING CALORIES: 309; TOTAL FAT: 13G; SATURATED FAT: 2G; PROTEIN: 43G; TOTAL CARBOHYDRATES: 5G; FIBER: 1G; CHOLESTEROL: 80MG; MACROS: FAT: 38%; PROTEIN: 56%; CARBS: 6%

LOBSTER ALFREDO

EASY, EGG-FREE, ONE-POT, QUICK PREP

SERVES 4 | PREP TIME: **5 MINUTES** | COOK TIME: **25 MINUTES**

Take your alfredo to the next level with this creamy, dreamy sauce featuring delicious morsels of lobster.

2 tablespoons extra-virgin olive oil

½ medium white onion, chopped

6 medium garlic cloves, minced

1 cup coconut cream

2 tablespoons ghee

1 tablespoon dried parsley

2 teaspoons dried basil

1 teaspoon dried oregano

½ teaspoon sea salt

1 pound shredded lobster meat

Zucchini Noodles (Zoodles, page 32)

Lemon wedges (optional)

1. Heat the olive oil in a large skillet over medium-high heat for 3 minutes or until the oil starts to shimmer.

2. Sauté the onion and garlic for 2 minutes or until the onion is translucent.

3. Whisk in the coconut cream, ghee, parsley, basil, oregano, and salt.

4. Cover, reduce the heat to low, and simmer for 15 minutes or until the sauce is reduced by half.

5. Add the lobster meat and cook for an additional 5 minutes or until the lobster is white and no longer translucent.

6. Serve over a bed of zoodles with a lemon wedge for squeezing (if using).

> **Variation Tip:** Have fun with this dish and swap out the lobster for crab meat or chicken.

PER SERVING CALORIES: 430; TOTAL FAT: 30G; SATURATED FAT: 21G; PROTEIN: 26G; TOTAL CARBOHYDRATES: 14G; FIBER: 3G; CHOLESTEROL: 182MG; MACROS: FAT: 63%; PROTEIN: 24%; CARBS: 13%

CAJUN CATFISH

SERVES 4 | PREP TIME: 5 MINUTES | COOK TIME: 20 MINUTES

Savor this blend of traditional Cajun spices that brings heat and flavor to tender catfish fillets!

1 tablespoon arrowroot flour

1 tablespoon ground paprika

1½ teaspoons dried oregano

1½ teaspoons dried thyme

1½ teaspoons ground cayenne pepper

½ teaspoon garlic powder

½ teaspoon ground white pepper

½ teaspoon freshly ground black pepper

½ teaspoon sea salt

1 tablespoon extra-virgin olive oil

4 (6-ounce) catfish fillets

1. Preheat the oven to 400°F. Line an edged baking sheet with parchment paper.

2. In a medium bowl, combine the arrowroot flour, paprika, oregano, thyme, cayenne, garlic powder, white pepper, black pepper, and salt.

3. Brush both sides of the catfish fillets with the olive oil, then coat them with the seasoning mix.

4. Bake the catfish fillets for 20 minutes or until the fish begins to flake. Serve immediately.

Variation Tip: Make extra seasoning and enjoy the Cajun flavors on all your favorite proteins.

PER SERVING CALORIES: 288; TOTAL FAT: 16G; SATURATED FAT: 5G; PROTEIN: 34G; TOTAL CARBOHYDRATES: 2G; FIBER: 1G; CHOLESTEROL: 99MG; MACROS: FAT: 50%; PROTEIN: 47%; CARBS: 3%

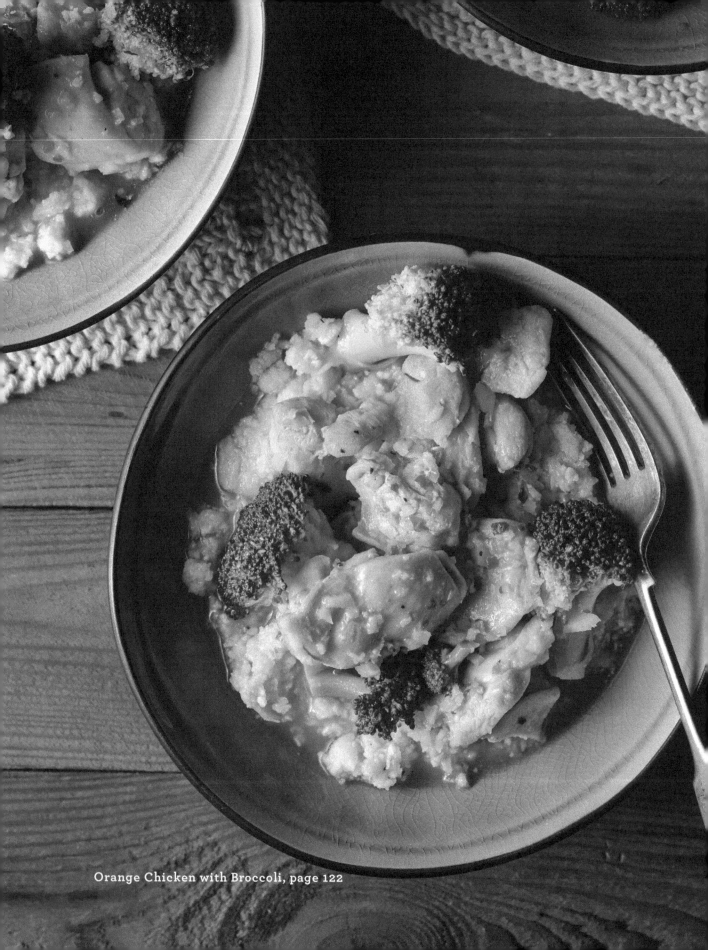

Orange Chicken with Broccoli, page 122

CHAPTER NINE

CHICKEN, TURKEY, DUCK, AND FOWL

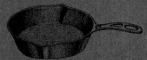

ORANGE CHICKEN WITH BROCCOLI

SERVES 4 | PREP TIME: 15 MINUTES | COOK TIME: 20 MINUTES

When I would order Chinese food, I'd always get my favorite, orange chicken and broccoli. I came up with this recipe because I wanted to make one of my favorite dishes into a healthy alternative that was easy enough for anyone to make.

3 tablespoons coconut oil

1 pound boneless and skinless chicken thighs, cut into 1-inch pieces

Sea salt

Freshly ground black pepper

⅓ cup freshly squeezed orange juice

4 medium garlic cloves, minced

1 tablespoon grated peeled fresh ginger

½ cup coconut aminos

6 tablespoons water

¼ teaspoon red pepper flakes

4 cups chopped broccoli florets

4 cups Grated Cauliflower Rice (page 37)

1. Heat the coconut oil in a large skillet over medium-high heat for 3 minutes or until the oil starts to shimmer.

2. Season the chicken pieces with salt and pepper.

3. Cook the chicken for 5 minutes or until partially browned with an opaque center. Remove the skillet from the heat and set aside.

4. In a small saucepan over medium-high heat, combine the orange juice, garlic, ginger, coconut aminos, water, and red pepper flakes. Bring to a boil. Cover, reduce the heat to low, and simmer for 5 minutes or until fragrant.

5. Meanwhile, fill a medium saucepan with 1 inch of water and bring to a boil. Carefully add the broccoli, cover, and reduce the heat to medium. Steam the broccoli for 5 minutes or until fork-tender. Drain.

6. Combine the sauce, steamed broccoli, and chicken.

7. Serve over Grated Cauliflower Rice.

Variation Tip: To limit the spice and make this an AIP-friendly dish, omit the red pepper flakes.

PER SERVING CALORIES: 331; TOTAL FAT: 15G; SATURATED FAT: 10G; PROTEIN: 27G; TOTAL CARBOHYDRATES: 22G; FIBER: 5G; CHOLESTEROL: 95MG; MACROS: FAT: 41%; PROTEIN: 33%; CARBS: 26%

ZESTY ITALIAN CHICKEN AND "RICE" CASSEROLE

AIP-FRIENDLY, ALLERGEN-FREE, EASY, EGG-FREE

SERVES 4 | PREP TIME: 15 MINUTES | COOK TIME: 55 MINUTES

Loaded with zesty Italian spices and a creamy sauce, this simple casserole is sure to please even the pickiest of eaters.

3 tablespoons extra-virgin olive oil, divided

2 medium celery stalks, chopped

½ medium white onion, diced

¼ cup cassava flour

1 cup full-fat coconut milk

2 cups water

1 pound boneless and skinless chicken breasts, cut into 1-inch pieces

2 tablespoons Zesty Italian Seasoning (page 232)

1 teaspoon sea salt

½ teaspoon freshly ground black pepper

1 tablespoon dried onion

1 teaspoon garlic powder

4 cups Grated Cauliflower Rice (page 37)

1. Preheat the oven to 325°F.

2. Heat 1½ tablespoons of olive oil in a medium sauce-pan over medium-high heat for 3 minutes or until the oil starts to shimmer.

3. Sauté the celery and onion for 3 minutes or until the onion is translucent.

4. Add the cassava flour and whisk for 1 minute or until smooth.

5. Slowly whisk in the coconut milk and water.

6. Cover and simmer on low for 10 minutes or until the sauce has thickened.

7. In a large bowl, combine the chicken with the remaining 1½ tablespoons of olive oil, the Italian seasoning, salt, pepper, dried onion, and garlic powder.

8. Assemble the casserole by layering the cauliflower rice, chicken, and sauce into an 8-by-8-inch baking dish.

9. Cover with aluminum foil and bake in the preheated oven for 40 minutes or until the cauliflower rice is tender and the chicken is no longer pink. Serve immediately.

Ingredient Tip: Swap out the coconut milk for an equal amount of almond milk.

PER SERVING CALORIES: 404; TOTAL FAT: 24G; SATURATED FAT: 12G; PROTEIN: 30G; TOTAL CARBOHYDRATES: 17G; FIBER: 4G; CHOLESTEROL: 65MG; MACROS: FAT: 53%; PROTEIN: 30%; CARBS: 17%

WHOLE ROASTED LEMON AND ROSEMARY CHICKEN

EGG-FREE, QUICK PREP

SERVES 4 TO 6 | PREP TIME: **10 MINUTES** | COOK TIME: **1 HOUR 10 MINUTES**

Relish this chicken's crispy outer skin and moist fall-off-the-bone meat with hints of lemon and rosemary throughout. To make this AIP-friendly chicken, prepare with coconut oil instead of grass-fed butter.

1 (3-pound) whole chicken

1 large lemon, sliced

4 large garlic
cloves, crushed

2 rosemary sprigs

2 tablespoons melted
grass-fed butter or
coconut oil

Sea salt

Freshly ground black pepper

1. Preheat the oven to 375°F.

2. Remove and discard the giblet bag from the chicken cavity, and pat dry.

3. Place the chicken, legs down, into a baking dish.

4. Stuff the chicken cavity with the lemon, garlic, and rosemary.

5. Brush the skin with the butter or coconut oil.

6. Season the chicken generously with salt and pepper.

7. Bake for 30 minutes. Using tongs, carefully flip the chicken so that the legs are up.

8. Bake for an additional 40 minutes or until the skin is browned and crisp and the chicken has an internal temperature of 165°F.

9. Remove the chicken from the oven and let it rest for 10 minutes before cutting and serving.

> **Accompaniment Tip:** Make Chicken Bone Broth (page 28) with the bones.

PER SERVING (6 OUNCES) CALORIES: 354; TOTAL FAT: 22G; SATURATED FAT: 8G; PROTEIN: 35G; TOTAL CARBOHYDRATES: 4G; FIBER: 0G; CHOLESTEROL: 43MG; MACROS: FAT: 56%; PROTEIN: 40%; CARBS: 4%

WHOLE HERB-ROASTED TURKEY

AIP-FRIENDLY, ALLERGEN-FREE, EGG-FREE, NUT-FREE, QUICK PREP

SERVES 6 TO 8 | PREP TIME: 10 MINUTES | COOK TIME: 1 HOUR 30 MINUTES

Whether you are roasting your first bird or celebrating Thanksgiving with family, this whole herb-roasted turkey will surely be a crowd-pleaser.

1 (6-pound) whole turkey with skin

1 cup chopped celery

1 cup chopped scallions, white and green parts

6 medium garlic cloves, chopped

¼ cup chopped fresh parsley

½ cup duck fat or lard, divided

2 tablespoons sea salt

¼ cup Chicken Bone Broth (page 28)

1. Preheat the oven to 325°F.

2. Remove and discard the giblet bag from the turkey cavity, and pat dry.

3. Place the turkey, legs up and wing tips tucked under the body, into a roasting pan.

4. In a food processor or blender, blend the celery, scallions, garlic, parsley, ¼ cup of duck fat, and salt on high for 1 minute or until smooth and green.

5. Run one hand between the skin and the meat of the turkey to loosen. Using your hand, rub the paste between the skin and meat, covering all surfaces.

6. In a small bowl, melt the remaining ¼ cup of duck fat in the microwave for 30 seconds or until melted completely. Whisk in the bone broth and brush the mixture onto the skin of the turkey. Reserve the rest for basting.

7. Cover the turkey with aluminum foil and bake for 1 hour, basting every 30 minutes.

8. Uncover the turkey and cook for 30 more minutes or until the skin is golden brown and crisp and the turkey has an internal temperature of 165°F.

9. Remove the turkey from the oven and let it rest for 20 minutes before cutting and serving.

> **Prep Tip:** For larger turkeys, cook for an additional 15 minutes per pound.

PER SERVING (6 OUNCES) CALORIES: 289; TOTAL FAT: 17G; SATURATED FAT: 6G; PROTEIN: 32G; TOTAL CARBOHYDRATES: 2G; FIBER: 0G; CHOLESTEROL: 113MG; MACROS: FAT: 53%; PROTEIN: 44%; CARBS: 3%

WILD PHEASANT IN MUSHROOM GRAVY

ALLERGEN-FREE, EASY, EGG-FREE, NUT-FREE

SERVES 2 | PREP TIME: **15 MINUTES** | COOK TIME: **45 MINUTES**

This lovely pheasant dinner is immersed in a mushroom gravy and topped with fresh parsley. If pheasant isn't available, swap in equal-sized duck or chicken breasts.

---

5 tablespoons extra-virgin olive oil, divided

2 (6-ounce) pheasant breasts

Sea salt

Freshly ground black pepper

1 cup chopped white onion

5 medium garlic cloves, minced

3 cups cremini or baby bella mushrooms, cut into ¼-inch-thick slices

1 cup white wine

2 tablespoons arrowroot flour

2 tablespoons water

1 cup Chicken Bone Broth (page 28)

¼ cup finely chopped fresh parsley (optional)

1. Heat 2 tablespoons of olive oil in a Dutch oven or stockpot over medium-high heat for 3 minutes or until the oil starts to shimmer.

2. Brush 1 tablespoon of olive oil onto the pheasant breasts. Season with salt and pepper.

3. Place the pheasant breasts into the Dutch oven and sear for 2 minutes, then flip and sear for an additional 2 minutes or until lightly browned but not cooked. Remove the pheasant and set aside.

4. Heat the remaining 2 tablespoons of olive oil in the Dutch oven over medium-high heat for 3 minutes or until the oil starts to shimmer.

5. Sauté the onion and garlic for 3 minutes or until fragrant and soft. Add the mushrooms and sauté for 3 minutes or until fork-tender. Add the white wine and cook for 5 minutes or until the liquid has reduced by half.

6. In a small bowl, whisk together the arrowroot flour and water. Pour into the Dutch oven.

7. Place the pheasant breasts into the Dutch oven and pour the broth over them.

8. Cover and reduce the heat to low. Simmer for 20 minutes or until the pheasant breasts are cooked through and have an internal temperature of 165°F.

9. Top with parsley (if using) and serve.

PER SERVING CALORIES: 634; TOTAL FAT: 42G; SATURATED FAT: 7G; PROTEIN: 48G; TOTAL CARBOHYDRATES: 16G; FIBER: 3G; CHOLESTEROL: 111MG; MACROS: FAT: 60%; PROTEIN: 30%; CARBS: 10%

CRISPY BAKED CHICKEN THIGHS

SERVES 4 | PREP TIME: **5 MINUTES** | COOK TIME: **30 MINUTES**

Savor the flavors of the paprika, thyme, garlic, and other spices in each comforting bite of these moist chicken thighs.

8 (4-ounce) skin-on and bone-in chicken thighs

1 tablespoon extra-virgin olive oil

1 teaspoon garlic powder

1 teaspoon onion powder

1 teaspoon ground paprika

1 teaspoon dried thyme

1 teaspoon dried oregano

1 teaspoon sea salt

1 teaspoon freshly ground black pepper

1. Preheat the oven to 425°F. Line an edged baking sheet with aluminum foil and top with an oven-safe wire rack.

2. Place the chicken onto the wire rack, skin-side up, in a single layer.

3. Brush the skin with the olive oil.

4. In a small bowl, combine the garlic powder, onion powder, paprika, thyme, oregano, salt, and pepper.

5. Use the seasoning mix to season the chicken skin generously.

6. Bake for 30 minutes or until the thighs have a crispy outer layer and an internal temperature of 165°F. Serve immediately.

Ingredient Tip: Use leftover meat from this recipe to make Chicken Potpie (page 134).

PER SERVING CALORIES: 339; TOTAL FAT: 23G; SATURATED FAT: 6G; PROTEIN: 31G; TOTAL CARBOHYDRATES: 2G; FIBER: 1G; CHOLESTEROL: 139MG; MACROS: FAT: 61%; PROTEIN: 37%; CARBS: 2%

BARBECUE CHICKEN AND PINEAPPLE

ALLERGEN-FREE, EGG-FREE, NUT-FREE, QUICK PREP

SERVES 4 | PREP TIME: **5 MINUTES** | COOK TIME: **6 HOURS**

Enjoy moist and juicy chicken breasts smothered in a simple, flavorful barbecue sauce with a side of fresh, sweet pineapple.

4 (4-ounce) boneless and skinless chicken breasts

1 teaspoon sea salt

1 teaspoon freshly ground black pepper

1 large red onion, cut into ½-inch-thick slices

2 cups Date-Infused Barbecue Sauce (page 237)

1 pineapple, peeled, cored, and sliced

1. Place the chicken breasts into a 6-quart or larger slow cooker. Season with salt and pepper.

2. Top with the onion and barbecue sauce.

3. Cover and cook on low for 6 hours or until the chicken is fork-tender.

4. Using two forks, shred the chicken in the slow cooker. Allow the chicken to marinate in the barbecue sauce for an additional 20 minutes.

5. Serve with pineapple slices.

> Ingredient Tip: If you're short on time, there are a variety of paleo-approved barbecue sauces that can be found at most health grocers.

PER SERVING CALORIES: 470; TOTAL FAT: 2G; SATURATED FAT: 0G; PROTEIN: 31G; TOTAL CARBOHYDRATES: 82G; FIBER: 11G; CHOLESTEROL: 65MG; MACROS: FAT: 4%; PROTEIN: 26%; CARBS: 70%

APRICOT GLAZED CHICKEN WINGS

ALLERGEN-FREE, EASY, EGG-FREE, NUT-FREE

SERVES 4 | PREP TIME: **20 MINUTES** | COOK TIME: **1 HOUR**

A deliciously sweet apricot glaze perfectly coats each chicken wing to create a beautiful caramelized texture and taste in this recipe.

¾ cup water

½ cup dried apricots

2 tablespoons raw honey

Juice of 1 lime

Zest of 1 lime

1 garlic clove, minced

1 teaspoon ground ginger

1 teaspoon chili powder

¼ teaspoon ground allspice

½ teaspoon sea salt

2 pounds chicken wings

1. In a small saucepan, bring the water to a gentle boil over medium-high heat.

2. Remove the saucepan from the heat. Put the apricots in the pot. Let them soak for 10 minutes or until fork-tender.

3. In a blender, combine the apricots, soaking water, honey, lime juice, lime zest, garlic, ginger, chili powder, allspice, and salt. Blend on high for 1 minute or until thick and smooth.

4. Preheat the oven to 350°F. Line a baking sheet with parchment paper.

5. In a large bowl, combine the chicken wings and apricot glaze until each wing is well coated.

6. Place the glazed chicken wings onto the prepared baking sheet in a single layer and bake for 30 minutes.

7. Flip the wings and cook for an additional 30 minutes or until the outer skins are crisp and the internal temperature is 165°F. Serve immediately.

> **Variation Tip:** The raw honey can be swapped out for an equal amount of maple syrup.

PER SERVING CALORIES: 584; TOTAL FAT: 36G; SATURATED FAT: 10G; PROTEIN: 43G; TOTAL CARBOHYDRATES: 22G; FIBER: 2G; CHOLESTEROL: 17MG; MACROS: FAT: 55%; PROTEIN: 29%; CARBS: 16%

SWEET AND SPICY CHICKEN SKEWERS

ALLERGEN-FREE, EASY, EGG-FREE, NUT-FREE, QUICK PREP, UNDER 30 MINUTES

SERVES 4 | PREP TIME: **10 MINUTES** | COOK TIME: **15 MINUTES**

In this satisfying dish, honey brings the sweetness while the red pepper flakes bring the heat. This tasty take on chicken skewers is sure to please.

---

1 large sweet potato, peeled and cut into 1-inch pieces

3 tablespoons extra-virgin olive oil

2 teaspoons garlic powder

2 teaspoons chili powder

1 teaspoon sea salt

1 teaspoon freshly ground black pepper

1 teaspoon ground cumin

1 teaspoon ground paprika

1 teaspoon red pepper flakes

6 tablespoons raw honey

2 tablespoons apple cider vinegar

2 (4-ounce) boneless and skinless chicken thighs, cut into 2-inch pieces

1 large red onion, quartered

1. In a medium stockpot, cover the sweet potatoes with water. Bring to a boil and cook over medium-high heat for 5 minutes (sweet potatoes will be only partially cooked).

2. Drain the sweet potatoes and set aside.

3. In a small bowl, whisk together the olive oil, garlic powder, chili powder, salt, pepper, cumin, paprika, red pepper flakes, honey, and apple cider vinegar. If using wooden skewers, start soaking them in water.

4. In a medium bowl, combine the chicken, sweet potatoes, onion, and dressing.

5. Preheat the grill to medium heat (about 350°F) or heat a cast iron skillet over medium-high heat.

6. Thread the skewers by alternating chicken, sweet potatoes, and onion until all the ingredients are used.

7. Grill the skewers on the preheated grill over indirect heat or in the cast iron skillet for 8 minutes or until the chicken is opaque in the center, turning every minute to avoid burning. Serve immediately.

Variation Tip: If you don't have boneless, skinless chicken thighs, use boneless, skinless chicken breasts instead.

PER SERVING CALORIES: 337; TOTAL FAT: 13G; SATURATED FAT: 2G; PROTEIN: 13G; TOTAL CARBOHYDRATES: 42G; FIBER: 4G; CHOLESTEROL: 48MG; MACROS: FAT: 35%; PROTEIN: 15%; CARBS: 50%

CHIMICHURRI BAKED CHICKEN BREAST

ALLERGEN-FREE, EASY, EGG-FREE, NUT-FREE

SERVES 4 | PREP TIME: **15 MINUTES, PLUS 15 MINUTES TO MARINATE** | COOK TIME: **15 MINUTES**

Say goodbye to dry chicken and hello to this perfectly baked chicken breast covered in a flavorful chimichurri sauce.

4 cups warm water

¼ cup sea salt, plus more
for seasoning

4 (4-ounce) boneless and
skinless chicken breasts

1 tablespoon extra-virgin
olive oil

Freshly ground black pepper

Chimichurri Sauce
(page 241)

1. In a large bowl, combine the water and ¼ cup of sea salt to make a brine. Stir until the salt has dissolved.

2. Put the chicken in the bowl to brine for 15 minutes.

3. Meanwhile, preheat the oven to 450°F.

4. Remove the chicken from the brine, and pat dry.

5. Place the chicken into a large baking dish in a single layer.

6. Brush with the olive oil and season with salt and pepper.

7. Bake for 15 minutes or until the chicken has an opaque center.

8. Remove from the oven and let rest for 5 minutes before slicing and serving with chimichurri sauce.

> **Make-Ahead Tip:** For extra moist and tender meat, brine your chicken in advance for up to 24 hours.

PER SERVING CALORIES: 216; TOTAL FAT: 12G; SATURATED FAT: 2G; PROTEIN: 26G; TOTAL CARBOHYDRATES: 1G; FIBER: 0G; CHOLESTEROL: 65MG; MACROS: FAT: 50%; PROTEIN: 48%; CARBS: 2%

CREAMY TURKEY AND SPAGHETTI SQUASH CASSEROLE

EASY

SERVES 4 | PREP TIME: 15 MINUTES | COOK TIME: 20 MINUTES

In this recipe, spaghetti squash and Italian seasoned ground turkey are coated in a delicious, creamy coconut-based sauce with hints of basil and oregano. This Italian-inspired meal is great to make for new moms or large families!

1 tablespoon extra-virgin olive oil

1 cup chopped white onion

6 garlic cloves, minced

1 pound ground turkey

1 cup full-fat coconut milk

1 medium egg

1 tablespoon Zesty Italian Seasoning (page 232)

1 teaspoon sea salt

1 teaspoon freshly ground black pepper

1 teaspoon garlic powder

1 medium or large spaghetti squash, cooked and shredded

1. Heat the olive oil in a large skillet over medium-high heat for 3 minutes or until the oil starts to shimmer.

2. Cook the onion, garlic, and turkey for 5 minutes or until the turkey is no longer pink.

3. Preheat the oven to 350°F.

4. In a small saucepan, whisk together the coconut milk, egg, Italian seasoning, salt, pepper, and garlic powder over medium heat for 5 minutes or until warmed.

5. To assemble the casserole, layer a 9-by-13-inch baking dish with spaghetti squash, turkey and vegetables, and sauce.

6. Bake uncovered for 10 minutes or until thoroughly warmed. Serve immediately.

Make-Ahead Tip: To cook the squash, cut it in half lengthwise, scrape the seeds out, lightly brush it with extra-virgin olive oil, and bake at 450°F for 30 minutes or until fork-tender.

PER SERVING CALORIES: 383; TOTAL FAT: 23G; SATURATED FAT: 12G; PROTEIN: 27G; TOTAL CARBOHYDRATES: 17G; FIBER: 1G; CHOLESTEROL: 41MG; MACROS: FAT: 54%; PROTEIN: 28%; CARBS: 18%

CREAMY WILD PHEASANT AND MUSHROOM STEW

AIP-FRIENDLY, ALLERGEN-FREE, EASY, EGG-FREE, QUICK PREP

SERVES 4 | PREP TIME: 10 MINUTES | COOK TIME: 6 HOURS

Relish moist and tender pheasant meat smothered in a delicious coconut-based sauce and complemented by earthy and toothsome mushrooms.

4 (6-ounce)
  pheasant breasts

1 teaspoon dried thyme

Sea salt

Freshly ground black pepper

6 ounces chopped cremini
  or baby bella mushrooms

½ large white
  onion, chopped

2 medium celery
  stalks, chopped

2 garlic cloves, minced

2 cups Chicken Bone Broth
  (page 28)

1 cup full-fat coconut milk

⅓ cup coconut aminos

3 tablespoons
  arrowroot flour

3 tablespoons warm water

1. Put the pheasant breasts into a 6-quart or larger slow cooker and season with the thyme, salt, and pepper.

2. Top with the mushrooms, onion, celery, and garlic.

3. Add the bone broth, coconut milk, and coconut aminos.

4. Cover and cook on low for 6 hours or until the pheasant is fork-tender.

5. Carefully remove the breasts from the slow cooker and shred the meat away from the bones. Return the meat to the slow cooker and discard the bones.

6. In a small bowl, whisk together the arrowroot flour and water for 30 seconds or until smooth. Add to the slow cooker and stir for 30 seconds. Cover and let set for 5 minutes or until the sauce has thickened, then serve.

Variation Tip: Pheasant can be replaced with chicken in this recipe.

PER SERVING CALORIES: 417; TOTAL FAT: 21G; SATURATED FAT: 15G; PROTEIN: 48G; TOTAL CARBOHYDRATES: 9G; FIBER: 3G; CHOLESTEROL: 112MG; MACROS: FAT: 45%; PROTEIN: 46%; CARBS: 9%

CHICKEN POTPIE

AIP-FRIENDLY, ALLERGEN-FREE, EASY, EGG-FREE, NUT-FREE

SERVES 4 | PREP TIME: 15 MINUTES | COOK TIME: 30 MINUTES

This recipe reimagines the traditional chicken potpie as a grain-free and dairy-free meal that the whole family will love.

1 tablespoon extra-virgin olive oil

3 small garlic cloves, minced

2 medium celery stalks, cut into ¼-inch-thick slices

1 large carrot, cut into ¼-inch-thick slices

½ large white onion, chopped

4 small cremini or baby bella mushrooms, chopped

2 tablespoons arrowroot flour

2 tablespoons warm water

¾ cup Chicken Bone Broth (page 28)

¼ teaspoon sea salt

½ teaspoon freshly ground black pepper

½ teaspoon dried thyme

2 cups chopped chicken breasts or thighs, cooked

2 cups Mashed Sweet Potatoes (page 34)

1. Preheat the oven to 350°F. Place a 9-inch pie dish on an aluminum foil–lined baking sheet.

2. Heat the olive oil in a large skillet over medium-high heat for 3 minutes or until the oil starts to shimmer.

3. Sauté the garlic, celery, carrot, onion, and mushrooms for 3 minutes or until the vegetables are soft.

4. In a small bowl, whisk together the arrowroot flour and water. Set aside.

5. Add the bone broth, salt, pepper, and thyme to the skillet and bring to a gentle boil.

6. Once boiling, remove the skillet from the heat and whisk in the arrowroot mixture for 30 seconds or until the sauce starts to thicken. Fold in the chopped chicken.

7. Pour the potpie filling into the prepared pie dish and cover with the mashed sweet potatoes, using a spatula to distribute them evenly.

8. Bake for 25 minutes or until the sauce starts to boil over. Let the potpie stand for 5 minutes before serving.

Make-Ahead Tip: If you have leftovers handy, use leftover chicken from Whole Roasted Lemon and Rosemary Chicken (page 124) or Crispy Baked Chicken Thighs (page 127).

PER SERVING CALORIES: 362; TOTAL FAT: 10G; SATURATED FAT: 2G; PROTEIN: 28G; TOTAL CARBOHYDRATES: 40G; FIBER: 5G; CHOLESTEROL: 59MG; MACROS: FAT: 25%; PROTEIN: 31%; CARBS: 44%

CRISPY CHICKEN TENDERS

EASY, QUICK PREP, UNDER 30 MINUTES

SERVES 4 | PREP TIME: **5 MINUTES** | COOK TIME: **10 MINUTES**

These tenders are coated with shredded coconut and tapioca flour to give them a delicious, crispy coating when fried in coconut oil.

1 cup coconut oil

½ cup tapioca flour

⅓ cup unsweetened shredded coconut

1 teaspoon ground paprika

¼ teaspoon sea salt

½ teaspoon freshly ground black pepper

1 large egg

1 pound chicken tenders

1. Heat the coconut oil in an 8-inch cast iron skillet over medium-high heat for 10 minutes or until the oil starts to shimmer.

2. In a medium bowl, combine the tapioca flour, coconut, paprika, salt, and pepper.

3. In a small bowl, whisk the egg.

4. Dredge the chicken tenders in the whisked egg and then in the flour mixture to coat. Shake off any excess flour.

5. Place the chicken tenders into the cast iron skillet in a single layer. Fry for 5 minutes, then flip and fry for an additional 5 minutes or until golden brown and crispy with an opaque center.

6. Transfer the chicken tenders to a paper towel–lined plate to remove excess oil before serving.

Accompaniment Tip: Whip up a honey mustard dipping sauce by whisking together 6 tablespoons of honey, 2 tablespoons of Dijon mustard, and 1 teaspoon of apple cider vinegar.

PER SERVING CALORIES: 301; TOTAL FAT: 17G; SATURATED FAT: 13G; PROTEIN: 28G; TOTAL CARBOHYDRATES: 9G; FIBER: 1G; CHOLESTEROL: 112MG; MACROS: FAT: 51%; PROTEIN: 37%; CARBS: 12%

WHOLE ROASTED DUCK

5 INGREDIENTS OR FEWER, EGG-FREE, QUICK PREP

SERVES 4 | PREP TIME: **10 MINUTES** | COOK TIME: **2 HOURS**

Delicious and browned to perfection, this duck with moist fall-off-the-bone meat is the perfect centerpiece for your table.

1 (6-pound) whole duck

½ cup melted grass-fed
   butter or coconut
   oil, divided

Sea salt

Freshly ground black pepper

1. Preheat the oven to 375°F. Remove the duck from its packaging, and pat dry.

2. Place the duck, breast-side up, into a roasting pan.

3. Brush ¼ cup of melted butter over the duck and season with salt and pepper.

4. Roast the duck for 1 hour.

5. Carefully pour the remaining ¼ cup of melted butter onto the duck. Rotate the pan and cook for an additional 1 hour or until browned and crisp. Let the duck rest for 10 minutes before cutting and serving.

Variation Tip: You can use a whole chicken instead of duck.

PER SERVING CALORIES: 578; TOTAL FAT: 50G; SATURATED FAT: 24G; PROTEIN: 32G; TOTAL CARBOHYDRATES: 0G; FIBER: 0G; CHOLESTEROL: 204MG; MACROS: FAT: 78%; PROTEIN: 22%; CARBS: 0%

ORANGE-ROSEMARY DUCK BREASTS

AIP-FRIENDLY, ALLERGEN-FREE, EGG-FREE, NUT-FREE, QUICK PREP, UNDER 30 MINUTES

SERVES 2 | PREP TIME: 10 MINUTES | COOK TIME: 15 MINUTES

This flavorful, tender, orange-rosemary duck brings restaurant quality home in an impressive yet easy meal.

2 (6-ounce) duck breasts

Sea salt

Freshly ground black pepper

1 tablespoon extra-virgin olive oil

½ cup freshly squeezed orange juice

5 rosemary sprigs

3 tablespoons raw honey

1. Preheat the oven to 400°F.

2. Slit the skin of the duck breasts in a crisscross pattern.

3. Season with salt and pepper.

4. Heat the olive oil in a cast iron skillet over medium heat for 10 minutes or until the oil starts to shimmer.

5. Place the duck breasts, skin-side down, into the skillet and cook for 8 minutes or until the duck starts to release its fat. Flip the breasts and cook for an additional 2 minutes or until golden brown and crisp.

6. Put the cast iron skillet directly into the preheated oven and cook for 5 minutes or until fork-tender and still slightly pink in the middle. Transfer the duck breasts from the skillet onto a cutting board and allow them to rest for 5 minutes.

7. Add the orange juice, rosemary, and honey to the duck fat and juices in the skillet and whisk for 30 seconds or until thickened.

8. Remove and discard the rosemary sprigs, pour the sauce over the duck breasts, and serve.

> Variation Tip: Chicken breasts or thighs also work well in this recipe.

PER SERVING CALORIES: 454; TOTAL FAT: 30G; SATURATED FAT: 10G; PROTEIN: 30G; TOTAL CARBOHYDRATES: 16G; FIBER: 0G; CHOLESTEROL: 136MG; MACROS: FAT: 59%; PROTEIN: 26%; CARBS: 15%

ASIAN-INSPIRED CHILI DUCK WINGS

ALLERGEN-FREE, EASY, EGG-FREE, NUT-FREE, QUICK PREP

SERVES 4 | PREP TIME: 10 MINUTES | COOK TIME: **2 HOURS 30 MINUTES**

This Asian-inspired dish is loaded with chiles that bring the spice and will not disappoint!

---

2 pounds duck wings

3 cups Chicken Bone Broth, more if needed (page 28)

2 large red chiles, seeded and roughly chopped

½ cup water

½ cup white wine vinegar

½ cup raw honey

1 teaspoon grated peeled fresh ginger

½ teaspoon sea salt

1. Place the duck wings into a Dutch oven or stockpot and pour in enough bone broth to cover them. (You may need more than 3 cups of broth depending on the size of the Dutch oven.)

2. Bring to a simmer over medium heat.

3. Cover and cook for 2 hours or until the meat is fork-tender and ready to split apart from the bone.

4. In a small saucepan, combine the chiles, water, white wine vinegar, honey, ginger, and salt. Cook over medium heat for 5 minutes or until fragrant.

5. Transfer the sauce to a food processor or blender and blend on high for 1 minute or until smooth and thick.

6. Preheat the oven to 425°F. Line an edged baking sheet with parchment paper or aluminum foil.

7. Reserve ¼ cup or more of the sauce for dipping. Then, in a large bowl, combine the duck wings and remaining sauce.

8. Place the wings onto the prepared baking sheet in a single layer and bake for 10 minutes. Flip and bake for an additional 10 minutes or until browned and crisp. Serve immediately.

> **Variation Tip:** Replace the red chiles with red or green jalapeños, or swap out the duck wings for chicken wings.

PER SERVING CALORIES: 394; TOTAL FAT: 10G; SATURATED FAT: 1G; PROTEIN: 39G; TOTAL CARBOHYDRATES: 37G; FIBER: 1G; CHOLESTEROL: 104MG; MACROS: FAT: 23%; PROTEIN: 40%; CARBS: 37%

SHREDDED JAMAICAN JERK CHICKEN WRAPS

ALLERGEN-FREE, EASY, EGG-FREE, QUICK PREP

SERVES 4 | PREP TIME: **5 MINUTES** | COOK TIME: **30 MINUTES**

The mangos in these wraps bring the spice down a notch so you can enjoy all the classic, tantalizing flavors of Jamaican jerk seasoning.

1 pound boneless and skinless chicken thighs

1 tablespoon extra-virgin olive oil

1 tablespoon chili powder

½ tablespoon garlic powder

1 teaspoon onion powder

1 teaspoon dried thyme

1 teaspoon ground paprika

1 teaspoon coconut sugar

½ teaspoon red pepper flakes

½ teaspoon ground allspice

¼ teaspoon ground nutmeg

¼ teaspoon freshly ground black pepper

¼ teaspoon sea salt

⅛ teaspoon ground cinnamon

1 head butter lettuce

1 medium mango, chopped

1. Preheat the oven to 425°F. Line an edged baking sheet with aluminum foil and top with an oven-safe wire rack.

2. Place the chicken, skin-side up, in a single layer onto the prepared wire rack. Brush the skin with the olive oil.

3. In a small bowl, combine the chili powder, garlic powder, onion powder, thyme, paprika, coconut sugar, red pepper flakes, allspice, nutmeg, pepper, salt, and cinnamon.

4. Season the chicken skin generously with the seasoning mix.

5. Bake the chicken for 30 minutes or until the thighs have a crispy outer layer and an internal temperature of 165°F.

6. In a large bowl, shred the chicken with two forks.

7. Wrap the shredded jerk chicken in a leaf of lettuce and top with mango before serving.

> **Make-Ahead Tip:** Make the jerk seasoning ahead of time in larger batches and keep it on hand for seasoning other meats and vegetables.

PER SERVING CALORIES: 253; TOTAL FAT: 9G; SATURATED FAT: 2G; PROTEIN: 24G; TOTAL CARBOHYDRATES: 19G; FIBER: 3G; CHOLESTEROL: 95MG; MACROS: FAT: 32%; PROTEIN: 38%; CARBS: 30%

TURKEY, SQUASH, AND APPLE HASH

AIP-FRIENDLY, ALLERGEN-FREE, EASY, EGG-FREE, NUT-FREE, ONE-POT, QUICK PREP

SERVES 4 | PREP TIME: 10 MINUTES | COOK TIME: **10 MINUTES**

Enjoy delicious notes of cinnamon and ginger mixed with sweet butternut squash in this one-skillet wonder meal.

---

2 tablespoons extra-virgin olive oil, divided

1 pound ground turkey

1 teaspoon dried thyme

1 teaspoon ground ginger

1 teaspoon ground cinnamon

1 teaspoon garlic powder

½ teaspoon ground turmeric

¼ teaspoon sea salt

½ teaspoon freshly ground black pepper

2 Gala apples, peeled, cored, and chopped

2 cups chopped butternut squash

1 medium white onion, chopped

2 cups baby spinach leaves

1. Heat 1 tablespoon of olive oil in a large skillet over medium-high heat for 3 minutes or until the oil starts to shimmer.

2. Cook the ground turkey, thyme, ginger, cinnamon, garlic powder, turmeric, salt, and pepper for 5 minutes or until the turkey is no longer pink.

3. Transfer the turkey to a plate and set aside.

4. In the skillet, heat the remaining 1 tablespoon of olive oil, and sauté the apples, butternut squash, and onion for 5 minutes or until the squash is fork-tender.

5. Add the spinach and stir for 20 to 30 seconds or until the spinach is partially wilted.

6. Transfer the ground turkey back into the skillet, stir to combine, and serve.

> **Variation Tip:** The butternut squash can be swapped out for sweet potatoes or any other winter squash as desired.

PER SERVING CALORIES: 325; TOTAL FAT: 17G; SATURATED FAT: 4G; PROTEIN: 22G; TOTAL CARBOHYDRATES: 21G; FIBER: 4G; CHOLESTEROL: 90MG; MACROS: FAT: 47%; PROTEIN: 27%; CARBS: 26%

BAJA CHICKEN FAJITAS

SERVES 4 | PREP TIME: **15 MINUTES** | COOK TIME: **10 MINUTES**

Savor the Mexican-inspired spices in these fajitas complemented by sweet onions and peppers.

---

2 pounds boneless and skinless chicken breast (5 to 6 breasts), cut into ¼-inch-thick slices

2 tablespoons freshly squeezed lime juice

1 teaspoon chili powder

1 teaspoon ground cumin

1 teaspoon garlic powder

1 teaspoon sea salt

1 teaspoon ground coriander

½ teaspoon freshly ground black pepper

2 tablespoons avocado oil

1 large white onion, cut into ¼-inch-thick slices

1 red bell pepper, cut into ½-inch-thick slices

1 yellow bell pepper, cut into ½-inch-thick slices

1 tablespoon chopped fresh cilantro

4 AIP/Allergen-Free Tortillas (page 36)

1 avocado, cut into ½-inch-thick slices

1. In a resealable quart-size bag, combine the chicken, lime juice, chili powder, cumin, garlic powder, salt, coriander, and pepper. Shake the bag to mix, coating the chicken well.

2. Heat the avocado oil in a cast iron skillet over medium-high heat for 5 minutes or until the oil starts to shimmer.

3. Transfer the chicken to the skillet and cook in a single layer for 2 minutes, then flip and cook for an additional 2 minutes or until the chicken is opaque. Transfer the chicken to a plate and set aside.

4. Return the skillet to the burner and sauté the onion and red and yellow bell peppers over medium-high heat for 5 minutes or until the onion is translucent.

5. Remove the skillet from the heat and stir in the chicken and cilantro.

6. Top the tortillas with the chicken, vegetables, and avocado. Serve.

> **Ingredient Tip:** Marinate the chicken overnight to save time and enjoy a more intense flavor.

PER SERVING CALORIES: 495; TOTAL FAT: 19G; SATURATED FAT: 4G; PROTEIN: 54G; TOTAL CARBOHYDRATES: 27G; FIBER: 7G; CHOLESTEROL: 130MG; MACROS: FAT: 35%; PROTEIN: 44%; CARBS: 21%

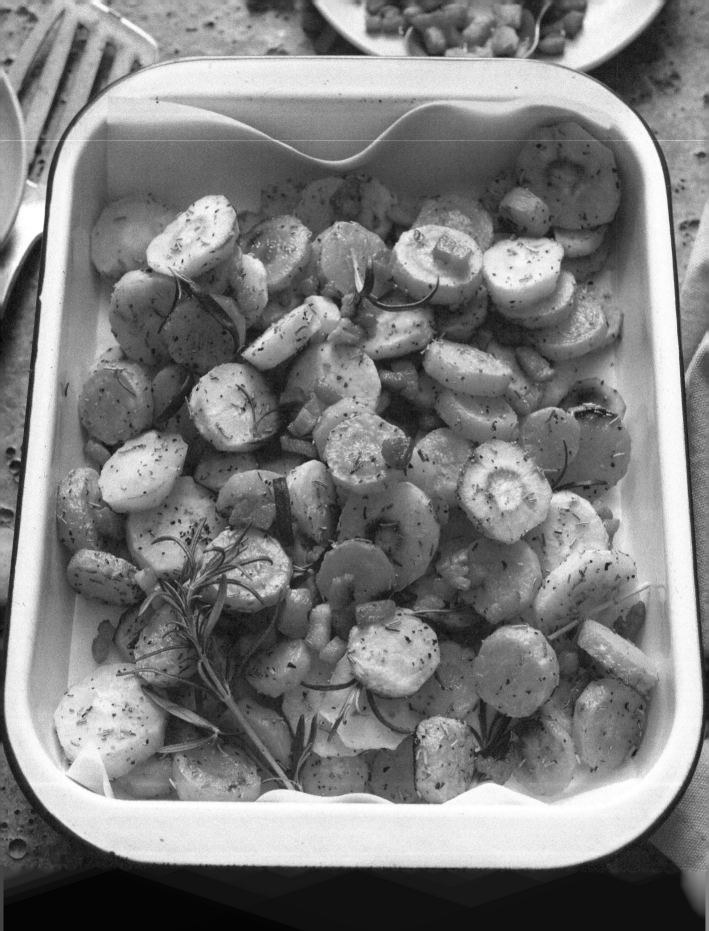

PORK

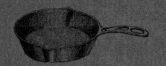

ROASTED ROOT VEGETABLES AND BACON

AIP-FRIENDLY, ALLERGEN-FREE, EGG-FREE, NUT-FREE, QUICK PREP

SERVES 4 | PREP TIME: 10 MINUTES | COOK TIME: 25 MINUTES

This sweet and savory root vegetable dish can be eaten as a side dish or as a main course.

4 parsnips, peeled and cut into ¼-inch-thick rounds

6 medium carrots, peeled and cut into ¼-inch-thick rounds

2 tablespoons extra-virgin olive oil

1 teaspoon dried rosemary

½ teaspoon freshly ground black pepper

1 pound nitrate- and sugar-free bacon, cooked and chopped

1. Preheat the oven to 425°F. Line an edged baking sheet with parchment paper.

2. In a large bowl, combine the parsnips, carrots, olive oil, rosemary, and pepper.

3. Arrange the vegetables in a single layer on the prepared baking sheet.

4. Cook for 25 minutes or until the vegetables are fork-tender and have a slightly browned crisp outside.

5. Remove from the oven, top with chopped bacon, and serve.

Ingredient Tip: Depending on the salt content of the bacon, you may or may not need to add salt to this dish.

PER SERVING CALORIES: 676; TOTAL FAT: 52G; SATURATED FAT: 16G; PROTEIN: 17G; TOTAL CARBOHYDRATES: 35G; FIBER: 9G; CHOLESTEROL: 77MG; MACROS: FAT: 69%; PROTEIN: 10%; CARBS: 21%

DRY-RUBBED RIBS

SERVES 4 | PREP TIME: **10 MINUTES** | COOK TIME: **2 HOURS**

These tender, fall-off-the-bone baby back ribs are slow cooked for 2 hours. They're delicious with any style of barbecue sauce.

---

3 pounds baby back ribs, membrane removed

¼ cup extra-virgin olive oil

¼ cup coconut sugar

2 teaspoons ground smoked paprika

2 teaspoons sea salt

2 teaspoons freshly ground black pepper

1 teaspoon ground mustard

1 teaspoon garlic powder

1 teaspoon onion powder

½ teaspoon celery salt

½ teaspoon ground cinnamon

¼ teaspoon cayenne pepper

1. Preheat the oven to 300°F. Line an edged baking sheet with parchment paper.

2. Put the ribs onto the prepared baking sheet and brush with the olive oil.

3. In a small bowl, combine the coconut sugar, paprika, salt, pepper, mustard, garlic powder, onion powder, celery salt, cinnamon, and cayenne.

4. Massage the ribs generously with the seasoning, coating evenly.

5. Bake for 2 hours or until the ribs are fork-tender with a crispy outer layer. Serve immediately.

Make-Ahead Tip: Make the seasoning ahead of time, or double the recipe and use it to season chicken or other proteins.

PER SERVING CALORIES: 740; TOTAL FAT: 48G; SATURATED FAT: 18G; PROTEIN: 51G; TOTAL CARBOHYDRATES: 26G; FIBER: 1G; CHOLESTEROL: 188MG; MACROS: FAT: 58%; PROTEIN: 28%; CARBS: 14%

PIZZA MEATBALLS WITH HOMEMADE MARINARA SAUCE

ALLERGEN-FREE, EASY, EGG-FREE

SERVES 4 | PREP TIME: **15 MINUTES** | COOK TIME: **30 MINUTES**

Satisfy your pizza craving with these bite-size meatballs dipped into a simple homemade marinara sauce.

FOR THE MARINARA SAUCE

- 2 tablespoons extra-virgin olive oil
- 2 medium garlic cloves, minced
- 1 (14-ounce) can fire-roasted diced tomatoes, drained
- 1 teaspoon coconut sugar
- ½ teaspoon sea salt
- ⅛ teaspoon freshly ground black pepper

FOR THE MEATBALLS

- 1 pound ground pork
- 8 slices uncured pepperoni, chopped
- ¼ cup nutritional yeast
- 1 tablespoon Zesty Italian Seasoning (page 232)
- 1 teaspoon coconut aminos
- ½ teaspoon sea salt
- ½ teaspoon freshly ground black pepper

TO MAKE THE MARINARA SAUCE

1. Heat the olive oil in a medium saucepan over medium heat for 3 minutes or until the oil starts to shimmer.

2. Sauté the garlic for 2 minutes or until golden brown and fragrant.

3. Add the tomatoes, coconut sugar, salt, and pepper. Stir to combine, then bring to a simmer.

4. Reduce the heat to low and simmer for 8 minutes or until the marinara has thickened. Remove from the heat and let cool for 10 minutes.

5. In a blender or food processor, blend the sauce for 30 seconds or until smooth.

TO MAKE THE MEATBALLS

1. Preheat the oven to 350°F. Line an edged baking sheet with aluminum foil and top with an oven-safe wire rack.

2. In a large bowl, combine the ground pork, pepperoni, nutritional yeast, Italian seasoning, coconut aminos, salt, and pepper.

3. Roll the mixture into 1½-inch balls and place on the prepared wire rack in a single layer.

4. Bake for 30 minutes or until the meatballs are cooked through and no longer pink in the middle.

5. Allow the meatballs to cool for 5 minutes before serving with homemade marinara.

> Ingredient Tip: Add more toppings to your pizza meatballs by folding in finely diced onions, bell peppers, mushrooms, or black olives.

PER SERVING CALORIES: 429; TOTAL FAT: 29G; SATURATED FAT: 9G; PROTEIN: 31G; TOTAL CARBOHYDRATES: 11G; FIBER: 5G; CHOLESTEROL: 363MG; MACROS: FAT: 61%; PROTEIN: 29%; CARBS: 10%

BACON-AND-APPLE-STUFFED PORK CHOPS

AIP-FRIENDLY, ALLERGEN-FREE, EGG-FREE, NUT-FREE, QUICK PREP

SERVES 4 | PREP TIME: **10 MINUTES** | COOK TIME: **30 MINUTES**

The sage enhances each bite of pork in this easy 40-minute recipe.

FOR THE FILLING

½ cup cooked chopped nitrate- and sugar-free bacon

¼ cup finely chopped white onion

1 medium Gala apple, peeled, cored, and finely chopped

4 small cremini or baby bella mushrooms, finely chopped

1 tablespoon dried sage

1 tablespoon extra-virgin olive oil

¼ teaspoon sea salt

FOR THE PORK CHOPS

1 tablespoon avocado oil

4 (6-ounce) bone-in pork chops, 2 inches thick

Sea salt

Freshly ground black pepper

TO MAKE THE FILLING

In a small bowl, combine the bacon, onion, apple, mushrooms, sage, olive oil, and salt. Set aside.

TO MAKE THE PORK CHOPS

1. Preheat the oven to 350°F. In a small bowl, cover 12 toothpicks with water.

2. Heat the avocado oil in a cast iron skillet over medium-high heat for 10 minutes or until the oil starts to shimmer.

3. Season the pork chops with salt and pepper. In each chop, slice the meat lengthwise without cutting through it, creating a pocket that is 2 inches deep and 3 inches wide.

4. Stuff each pork chop with some of the filling, reserving ¼ cup, then pinch each opening and skewer with 3 toothpicks to seal the filling in.

5. Sear the stuffed pork chops in the cast iron skillet for 4 minutes. Flip and sear for an additional 4 minutes or until the chops are crisp and brown.

6. Add the remaining ¼ cup of filling to the skillet, put the skillet in the oven, and bake for 20 minutes or until the internal temperature of the pork chops is 145°F. Let the pork chops rest 10 minutes before serving.

> **Variation Tip:** Swap out the sage with equal parts of dried rosemary or thyme.

PER SERVING CALORIES: 550; TOTAL FAT: 38G; SATURATED FAT: 12G; PROTEIN: 41G; TOTAL CARBOHYDRATES: 11G; FIBER: 2G; CHOLESTEROL: 80MG; MACROS: FAT: 62%; PROTEIN: 30%; CARBS: 8%

SHREDDED BARBECUE PORK

SERVES 4 | PREP TIME: **5 MINUTES** | COOK TIME: **6 HOURS**

Enjoy this moist, shredded pork over a baked sweet potato or on a bed of leafy greens.

3 pounds pork tenderloin

2 cups Date-Infused Barbecue Sauce (page 237)

1. Add the pork tenderloin into a 6-quart or larger slow cooker and cover with barbecue sauce.

2. Cover and cook on low for 6 hours or until the pork loin is fork-tender.

3. Using two forks, shred the pork in the slow cooker. Serve.

> **Ingredient Tip:** Double the Date-Infused Barbecue Sauce recipe on page 237 to have extra on hand for dipping.

PER SERVING CALORIES: 600; TOTAL FAT: 8G; SATURATED FAT: 0G; PROTEIN: 76G; TOTAL CARBOHYDRATES: 56G; FIBER: 8G; CHOLESTEROL: 225MG; MACROS: FAT: 12%; PROTEIN: 51%; CARBS: 37%

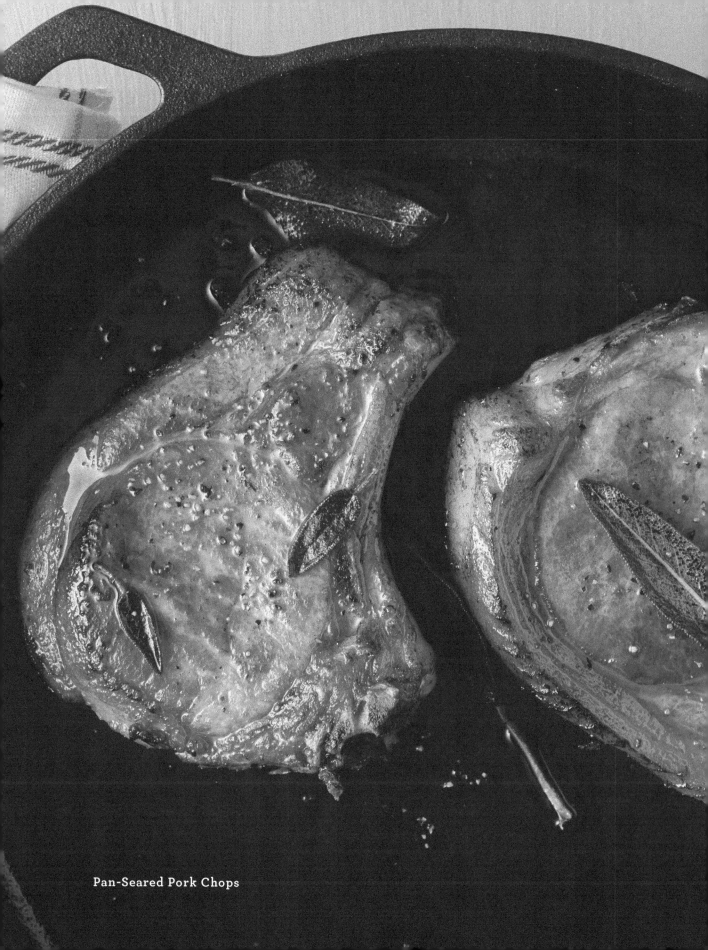

Pan-Seared Pork Chops

PAN-SEARED PORK CHOPS

SERVES 4 | PREP TIME: 5 MINUTES | COOK TIME: **10 MINUTES**

Don't let the lack of ingredients fool you—the secret to a perfectly mouthwatering pork chop lies in the cast iron skillet. If you like, garnish with crispy fried sage for extra flavor!

1 tablespoon avocado oil

4 (6-ounce) bone-in pork chops, 1 inch thick, close to room temperature

Sea salt

Freshly ground black pepper

1. Heat the avocado oil in a cast iron skillet over medium-high heat for 10 minutes or until the oil starts to shimmer.

2. Season the pork chops with salt and pepper.

3. Sear the pork chops for 5 minutes, then flip and sear for an additional 5 minutes or until the chops are crisp and brown.

4. Transfer to a cutting board and allow the pork chops to rest for 5 minutes before serving.

Accompaniment Tip: Serve with a side of Bacon-Roasted Brussels Sprouts (page 196), Cinnamon Sugar Applesauce (page 197), or Maple Acorn Squash (page 202).

PER SERVING CALORIES: 379; TOTAL FAT: 27G; SATURATED FAT: 8G; PROTEIN: 32G; TOTAL CARBOHYDRATES: 2G; FIBER: 0G; CHOLESTEROL: 59MG; MACROS: FAT: 64%; PROTEIN: 34%; CARBS: 2%

BLT WRAPS

SERVES 4 | PREP TIME: 10 MINUTES

Nothing beats the nutrition and taste of these BLT wraps. They're loaded with all the traditional ingredients but wrapped together in a grain-free wrap.

4 AIP/Allergen-Free Tortillas (page 36) or coconut wraps

Real Paleo Mayonnaise (page 234) or Creamy Ranch Dressing (page 236), for serving

8 nitrate- and sugar-free bacon slices, cooked

½ cup chopped lettuce

¼ cup diced Roma tomatoes

1 medium avocado, chopped

1. Layer each tortilla with the mayonnaise, 2 slices of bacon, lettuce, tomatoes, and avocado.

2. Roll and serve immediately.

> **Variation Tip:** Add your favorite nitrate- and sugar-free deli meat for extra protein.

PER SERVING CALORIES: 449; TOTAL FAT: 37G; SATURATED FAT: 8G; PROTEIN: 16G; TOTAL CARBOHYDRATES: 13G; FIBER: 4G; CHOLESTEROL: 54MG; MACROS: FAT: 74%; PROTEIN: 14%; CARBS: 12%

PORK FRIED "RICE"

SERVES 4 | PREP TIME: **10 MINUTES** | COOK TIME: **15 MINUTES**

Have your favorite restaurant-quality fried rice on the table in 30 minutes with this easy-to-assemble pork dish.

1 tablespoon avocado oil

1 pound ground pork

2 medium garlic cloves, minced

1 teaspoon ground ginger

3 tablespoons coconut aminos

1 cup shredded carrots

1 cup shredded cabbage

1 cup chopped scallions, white and green parts

4 cups Grated Cauliflower Rice (page 37)

3 large eggs

1. Heat the avocado oil in a large skillet over medium-high heat for 3 minutes or until the oil starts to shimmer.

2. Cook the pork, garlic, and ginger for 5 minutes or until the pork is no longer pink.

3. Add the coconut aminos, carrots, cabbage, scallions, and cauliflower rice. Cook for an additional 5 minutes, stirring occasionally, until the cauliflower rice is tender.

4. Push the contents in the skillet away from the middle to create an opening for the eggs. Crack the eggs into the center of the skillet and allow them to cook for 1 minute before scrambling with a wooden spoon. Serve immediately.

> Variation Tip: Swap out ground pork for ground beef to make beef fried "rice."

PER SERVING CALORIES: 375; TOTAL FAT: 23G; SATURATED FAT: 8G; PROTEIN: 28G; TOTAL CARBOHYDRATES: 14G; FIBER: 4G; CHOLESTEROL: 215MG; MACROS: FAT: 55%; PROTEIN: 30%; CARBS: 15%

SWEET AND SPICY PORK BELLY BITES

SERVES 8 | PREP TIME: 5 MINUTES, PLUS 30 MINUTES TO MARINATE | COOK TIME: **30 MINUTES**

These tender pork belly bites are packed full of lush flavors that will have you coming back for more.

¼ cup apple cider vinegar

¼ cup coconut sugar

½ teaspoon garlic powder

2 teaspoons tomato paste

1 teaspoon red
   pepper flakes

¼ teaspoon sea salt

1½ pounds pork belly, cut
   into 1-inch-thick slices

1. In a small saucepan, whisk together the apple cider vinegar, coconut sugar, garlic powder, tomato paste, red pepper flakes, and salt over medium heat for 5 minutes or until bubbles start to form. Remove from the heat and cool for 5 minutes.

2. Combine the pork belly slices and marinade in a resealable quart-size bag and shake to cover.

3. Let the pork marinate in the refrigerator for 30 minutes.

4. Preheat the oven to 425°F. Line an edged baking sheet with aluminum foil and top with an oven-safe wire rack.

5. Remove the marinated pork belly from the bag and place each piece on the prepared wire rack.

6. Cook for 15 minutes, then flip and cook for an additional 15 minutes or until a crispy, brown outer layer has formed. Let cool and serve.

> **Variation Tip:** Coconut sugar can be replaced with an equal amount of raw honey.

PER SERVING CALORIES: 469; TOTAL FAT: 45G; SATURATED FAT: 15G; PROTEIN: 9G; TOTAL CARBOHYDRATES: 7G; FIBER: 0G; CHOLESTEROL: 60MG; MACROS: FAT: 86%; PROTEIN: 8%; CARBS: 6%

KOREAN-STYLE PORK CHOPS

ALLERGEN-FREE, EASY, EGG-FREE, QUICK PREP

SERVES 4 | PREP TIME: **5 MINUTES, PLUS 20 MINUTES TO MARINATE** | COOK TIME: **20 MINUTES**
Juicy pork in a simple Korean-style marinade makes for the perfect weeknight dinner.

4 (6-ounce) boneless pork chops, ½ inch thick

2 tablespoons avocado oil, divided

¼ cup coconut aminos

1 tablespoon raw honey

2 medium garlic cloves, minced

1 teaspoon ground ginger

2 teaspoons paleo-approved hot sauce

1. Preheat the oven to 400°F.

2. In a resealable quart-size bag, combine the pork chops, 1 tablespoon of avocado oil, the coconut aminos, honey, garlic, ground ginger, and hot sauce. Let the pork marinate in the refrigerator for 20 minutes.

3. After 10 minutes, heat the remaining 1 tablespoon of avocado oil in a cast iron skillet over medium-high heat for 5 minutes or until the oil starts to shimmer.

4. Sear the pork chops for 5 minutes, then flip and cook for an additional 5 minutes or until the chops are crisp and brown.

5. Add the remaining marinade from the bag and put the skillet in the oven for 10 minutes or until the pork reaches an internal temperature of 145°F.

6. Transfer the pork chops to a cutting board and allow them to rest for 5 minutes, then serve.

Make-Ahead Tip: Marinate overnight for a more intense, punchier flavor.

PER SERVING CALORIES: 351; TOTAL FAT: 23G; SATURATED FAT: 7G; PROTEIN: 30G; TOTAL CARBOHYDRATES: 6G; FIBER: 0G; CHOLESTEROL: 66MG; MACROS: FAT: 59%; PROTEIN: 34%; CARBS: 7%

CUBAN BRAISED PORK SHOULDER

SERVES 4 | PREP TIME: **10 MINUTES, PLUS 24 HOURS TO MARINATE** | COOK TIME: **3 HOURS**

Enjoy this citrusy braised pork with robust garlic, parsley, and lots of carrots and onions.

3 pounds boneless
  pork shoulder

2 teaspoons sea salt

2 teaspoons freshly ground
  black pepper

5 medium garlic
  cloves, minced

2 scallions, white and green
  parts, chopped

¾ cup extra-virgin olive oil

½ cup chopped
  fresh parsley

2 tablespoons dried oregano

1½ teaspoons grated
  orange zest

1 teaspoon grated lime zest

1 teaspoon ground cumin

2 medium white onions, cut
  into 1-inch-thick slices

1 pound carrots, peeled
  and cut into
  ½-inch-thick spears

1. Put the pork shoulder in a Dutch oven or stockpot and season with the salt and pepper.

2. In a small bowl, muddle the garlic, scallions, olive oil, parsley, oregano, orange zest, lime zest, and cumin.

3. Rub the paste over the pork shoulder, covering all sides generously.

4. Top with the onions and carrots, cover, and marinate in the refrigerator for 24 hours.

5. When the pork is done marinating, preheat the oven to 350°F.

6. Put the Dutch oven into the oven and cook for 3 hours or until the meat is fork-tender and breaking apart.

7. Remove the Dutch oven and allow the meat to rest on the stovetop for 10 minutes before serving.

Make-Ahead Tip: You can prepare this dish the day before and pop it in the oven in time for lunch or dinner.

PER SERVING CALORIES: 1,287; TOTAL FAT: 107G; SATURATED FAT: 30G; PROTEIN: 60G; TOTAL CARBOHYDRATES: 21G; FIBER: 6G; CHOLESTEROL: 240MG; MACROS: FAT: 75%; PROTEIN: 19%; CARBS: 6%

HONEY-ORANGE GLAZED HAM

AIP-FRIENDLY, ALLERGEN-FREE, EASY, EGG-FREE

SERVES 8 | PREP TIME: **15 MINUTES** | COOK TIME: **4 HOURS**

This ham is perfect for the holidays, as it's unbelievably flavorful, tender, and aromatic.

FOR THE GLAZE

2 (4-inch) cinnamon sticks

2 oranges, cut into
⅛-inch-thick slices

2 cups freshly squeezed
orange juice

1 cup coconut oil

1 cup water

½ cup raw honey

¼ teaspoon ground cloves

FOR THE HAM

8 pounds uncured
sugar-free bone-in ham

¼ cup melted coconut oil

8 fresh sage leaves,
finely chopped

1 teaspoon sea salt

1 teaspoon freshly ground
black pepper

TO MAKE THE GLAZE

1. In a medium saucepan, combine the cinnamon sticks, orange slices, orange juice, coconut oil, water, honey, and cloves over medium heat.

2. Bring to a gentle boil, cover, and reduce the heat to low.

3. Allow the glaze to simmer for 30 minutes or until the liquid thickens. Set aside.

TO MAKE THE HAM

1. Preheat the oven to 300°F.

2. Put the ham, fatty-side up, into a roasting pan.

3. Score the ham with a sharp knife in a crisscross pattern.

4. In a small bowl, combine the coconut oil, sage, salt, and pepper and pour over the ham.

5. Bake the ham for 2 hours.

6. Pour the glaze over the ham and cook for an additional 2 hours, basting every 30 minutes, until the ham has a golden-brown glazed coating and reaches an internal temperature of 145°F.

7. Remove the ham from the oven and allow it to rest for 10 minutes before slicing and serving.

> **Ingredient Tip:** At your butcher or grocery store, look for quality local ham that is minimally processed and sugar-free.

PER SERVING CALORIES: 1,405; TOTAL FAT: 117G; SATURATED FAT: 50G; PROTEIN: 76G; TOTAL CARBOHYDRATES: 12G; FIBER: 0G; CHOLESTEROL: 300MG; MACROS: FAT: 75%; PROTEIN: 22%; CARBS: 3%

GARLIC AND HERB PORK TENDERLOIN

ALLERGEN-FREE, EASY, EGG-FREE, NUT-FREE, ONE-POT, QUICK PREP, UNDER 30 MINUTES

SERVES 4 | PREP TIME: **5 MINUTES** | COOK TIME: **20 MINUTES**

Perfectly seasoned and delicious, this garlic and herb pork pairs well with Bacon-Roasted Brussels Sprouts (page 196) and Cinnamon Sugar Applesauce (page 197).

---

3 pounds pork tenderloin

**4 large garlic
   cloves, minced**

**2 tablespoons extra-virgin
   olive oil**

1 teaspoon dried sage

1 teaspoon dried oregano

1 teaspoon dried thyme

1 teaspoon onion powder

1½ teaspoons sea salt

**½ teaspoon freshly ground
   black pepper**

**½ teaspoon red
   pepper flakes**

1. Preheat the oven to 400°F.

2. Put the tenderloin in an 8-by-8-inch or larger baking dish.

3. In a small bowl, combine the garlic, olive oil, sage, oregano, thyme, onion powder, salt, pepper, and red pepper flakes to form a paste.

4. Generously spread the paste over the pork loin, covering it evenly.

5. Cook for 20 minutes or until the internal temperature reaches 145°F.

6. Transfer the pork to a cutting board and allow it to rest for 10 minutes before cutting and serving.

> Make-Ahead Tip: Marinate the pork in the refrigerator the night before to save time on prep.

PER SERVING CALORIES: 431; TOTAL FAT: 15G; SATURATED FAT: 4G; PROTEIN: 72G; TOTAL CARBOHYDRATES: 2G; FIBER: 1G; CHOLESTEROL: 225MG; MACROS: FAT: 31%; PROTEIN: 67%; CARBS: 2%

BACON-WRAPPED PINEAPPLE BITES

5 INGREDIENTS OR FEWER, ALLERGEN-FREE, EGG-FREE, QUICK PREP

MAKES 16 TO 18 BITES | PREP TIME: **10 MINUTES** | COOK TIME: **20 MINUTES**

Bacon pairs well with just about everything, including the sweet, aromatic flavors of fresh pineapple and coconut sugar.

½ pineapple, peeled, cored, and cut into 1-inch cubes

1 tablespoon coconut sugar

1 tablespoon coconut aminos

1 pound nitrate- and sugar-free bacon

Date-Infused Barbecue Sauce (page 237), for serving

1. Preheat the oven to 425°F. Line an edged baking sheet with aluminum foil and top with an oven-safe wire rack. In a small bowl, soak 16 to 18 toothpicks in water.

2. In a large bowl, combine the pineapple, coconut sugar, and coconut aminos.

3. Cut the bacon in half. Wrap each pineapple piece with bacon and secure with a toothpick. Place the bacon-wrapped pineapple bites on the prepared wire rack.

4. Cook for 8 minutes, then carefully flip and bake for an additional 8 to 10 minutes or until the bacon has browned and is slightly crispy. For crispier bacon, turn the broiler on high for 2 minutes, but watch the bacon to avoiding burning it.

5. Remove from the oven and cool before serving with barbecue sauce.

> **Variation Tip:** Coconut sugar can be replaced with raw honey.

PER SERVING (2 BITES) CALORIES: 296; TOTAL FAT: 16G; SATURATED FAT: 5G; PROTEIN: 16G; TOTAL CARBOHYDRATES: 22G; FIBER: 3G; CHOLESTEROL: 42MG; MACROS: FAT: 49%; PROTEIN: 21%; CARBS: 30%

CRISPY PORK CUTLETS

SERVES 4 | PREP TIME: **5 MINUTES** | COOK TIME: **15 MINUTES**

These crispy pork cutlets have a crunchy outer layer that surrounds moist, tender meat. The tasty breading features robust spices such as garlic, paprika, and freshly ground pepper.

2 tablespoons avocado oil

½ cup blanched almond flour (page 29)

2 tablespoons arrowroot flour

1 teaspoon sea salt

1 teaspoon freshly ground black pepper

1 teaspoon garlic powder

½ teaspoon ground paprika

2 large eggs

4 (4-ounce) pork cutlets, ¼ inch thick

1. Preheat the oven to 450°F.

2. Heat the avocado oil in a cast iron skillet over medium-high heat for 10 minutes or until the oil starts to shimmer.

3. In a medium bowl, combine the almond flour, arrowroot flour, salt, pepper, garlic powder, and paprika.

4. In another medium bowl, whisk the eggs.

5. Dip each pork cutlet into the eggs, then dredge each one in the flour mixture.

6. Carefully place the cutlets in the skillet, sear for 2 minutes, then flip and sear for an additional 2 minutes or until both sides have a crispy, golden layer.

7. Put the skillet directly into the preheated oven and cook for 8 minutes or until the pork reaches an internal temperature of 140°F. Let the cutlets rest for 10 minutes before serving.

> **Prep Tip:** If you can't find ¼-inch-thick pork cutlets, place the cutlets between two sheets of parchment paper or wax paper and pound them down using a meat mallet, heavy rolling pin, or cast iron skillet.

PER SERVING CALORIES: 294; TOTAL FAT: 17G; SATURATED FAT: 3G; PROTEIN: 31G; TOTAL CARBOHYDRATES: 4G; FIBER: 1G; CHOLESTEROL: 148MG; MACROS: FAT: 52%; PROTEIN: 42%; CARBS: 6%

PORK CARNITAS

ALLERGEN-FREE, EASY, EGG-FREE, NUT-FREE, QUICK PREP

SERVES 4 | PREP TIME: 10 MINUTES | COOK TIME: 8 HOURS

Any night of the week is a good night to enjoy the authentic flavors of this tender pork married with cumin, oregano, onion, and zippy jalapeño.

FOR THE SPICE PASTE

1 tablespoon extra-virgin olive oil

1 tablespoon dried oregano

2 teaspoons ground cumin

1 teaspoon sea salt

1 teaspoon freshly ground black pepper

FOR THE PORK

2 pounds pork shoulder

1 small white onion, chopped

1 medium jalapeño, chopped

4 medium garlic cloves, minced

¾ cup freshly squeezed orange juice

4 AIP/Allergen-Free Tortillas (page 36)

TO MAKE THE SPICE PASTE

In a small bowl, make the paste by combining the olive oil, oregano, cumin, salt, and pepper. Stir to combine thoroughly.

TO MAKE THE PORK

1. Put the pork shoulder into a 6-quart or larger slow cooker.

2. Generously spread the paste over the pork shoulder, covering it evenly. Top with the onion, jalapeño, garlic, and orange juice.

3. Cover and cook on low for 8 hours or until the meat is fork-tender.

4. Shred the pork with two forks in the slow cooker, wrap in the tortillas, and serve.

Make-Ahead Tip: To save time, make the tortillas the night before.

PER SERVING CALORIES: 704; TOTAL FAT: 52G; SATURATED FAT: 19G; PROTEIN: 39G; TOTAL CARBOHYDRATES: 20G; FIBER: 3G; CHOLESTEROL: 160MG; MACROS: FAT: 66%; PROTEIN: 22%; CARBS: 12%

SPICY PORK BOWL

ALLERGEN-FREE, EASY, EGG-FREE, NUT-FREE, QUICK PREP

SERVES 4 | PREP TIME: **10 MINUTES** | COOK TIME: **6 HOURS**

This spicy pork bowl is a Korean-inspired dish that's packed full of deliciously addictive spicy flavors.

3 pounds pork shoulder

¾ cup apple cider vinegar

½ cup Dijon mustard

¼ cup Sugar-Free Ketchup (page 235)

2 medium garlic cloves, minced

1 teaspoon cayenne pepper

1 teaspoon sea salt

½ teaspoon freshly ground black pepper

4 cups Grated Cauliflower Rice (page 37)

4 scallions, white and green parts, chopped

1. Put the pork shoulder in a 6-quart or larger slow cooker.

2. In a medium saucepan, whisk together the apple cider vinegar, mustard, ketchup, garlic, cayenne, salt, and pepper over medium heat for 5 minutes or until the sauce becomes thick and fragrant.

3. Pour the sauce over the pork and cover.

4. Cook on low for 6 hours or until the pork is fork-tender with an internal temperature of 145°F.

5. Using two forks, shred the pork in the slow cooker. Serve over a bowl of cauliflower rice and top with scallions.

Ingredient Tip: Cut back on the cayenne pepper for a less spicy dish, or for more spice, add more.

PER SERVING CALORIES: 910; TOTAL FAT: 70G; SATURATED FAT: 24G; PROTEIN: 61G; TOTAL CARBOHYDRATES: 9G; FIBER: 4G; CHOLESTEROL: 240MG; MACROS: FAT: 69%; PROTEIN: 27%; CARBS: 4%

PORK MARBELLA

AIP-FRIENDLY, ALLERGEN-FREE, EASY, EGG-FREE, ONE-POT, QUICK PREP

SERVES 4 | PREP TIME: 10 MINUTES, PLUS 2 HOURS TO MARINATE | COOK TIME: 35 MINUTES

This dish has all the flavor of a restaurant-quality chicken marbella, but it's made with luscious pork tenderloin instead!

2 pounds pork tenderloin

½ cup dates, pitted and chopped

½ cup Spanish green olives, pitted

⅓ cup coconut sugar

¼ cup extra-virgin olive oil

¼ cup capers plus 1 tablespoon caper liquid

¼ cup red wine vinegar

4 garlic cloves, minced

2 bay leaves

1 tablespoon dried oregano

2 teaspoons sea salt

1 tablespoon coconut oil

¼ cup chopped fresh parsley

1. In a resealable quart-size bag, combine the pork, dates, olives, coconut sugar, olive oil, capers and liquid, red wine vinegar, garlic, bay leaves, oregano, and salt. Set in the refrigerator to marinate for 2 hours.

2. A few minutes before the pork is finished marinating, preheat the oven to 350°F.

3. Heat a cast iron skillet over medium-high heat for 10 minutes or until the oil starts to shimmer.

4. Remove the marinated tenderloin from the bag. Sear it in the cast iron skillet for 2 minutes, then flip and sear for an additional 2 minutes or until it's crisp and brown.

5. Pour the remaining marinade into the cast iron skillet and put it in the oven for 10 minutes.

6. Flip the tenderloin and baste. Cook for an additional 10 to 15 minutes or until the pork is no longer pink and has an internal temperature of 145°F. Transfer the pork to a cutting board and allow it to rest for 10 minutes before cutting.

7. Meanwhile, return the cast iron skillet with the drippings to the stove over medium-high heat. Add the coconut oil and whisk for 5 minutes or until the marinade has slightly reduced.

8. Add the parsley, pour the marinade over the pork, and serve.

Make-Ahead Tip: Marinate the pork overnight to save time on dinner prep.

PER SERVING CALORIES: 542; TOTAL FAT: 22G; SATURATED FAT: 7G; PROTEIN: 49G; TOTAL CARBOHYDRATES: 37G; FIBER: 2G; CHOLESTEROL: 150MG; MACROS: FAT: 37%; PROTEIN: 36%; CARBS: 27%

PORK CHILI VERDE

ALLERGEN-FREE, EASY, EGG-FREE, NUT-FREE

SERVES 4 TO 6 | PREP TIME: 20 MINUTES, PLUS 4 HOURS TO MARINATE |
COOK TIME: 6 HOURS 5 MINUTES

This recipe takes your zingy tomatillo- and serrano-tinged chili to the next level. Serve it over a bed of Grated Cauliflower Rice (page 37) or folded into an AIP/Allergen-Free Tortilla (page 36).

FOR THE MARINADE

2 pounds pork stew meat

6 medium garlic cloves, minced

½ cup apple cider vinegar

½ cup dry white wine

½ cup avocado oil

⅓ cup chopped cilantro

Juice of 1 lime

Zest of 1 lime

2 tablespoons ground cumin

1 tablespoon whole peppercorns

1 tablespoon dried oregano

1 teaspoon sea salt

FOR THE CHILI VERDE

1½ pounds tomatillos, husked and rinsed

2 medium serrano peppers

1 garlic clove, peeled

½ large white onion, cut into 1-inch-thick slices

1 cup Chicken Bone Broth (page 28)

2 tablespoons chopped fresh cilantro

⅛ teaspoon ground fennel

½ teaspoon sea salt

TO MAKE THE MARINADE

1. In a resealable quart-size bag, combine the pork, garlic, apple cider vinegar, white wine, avocado oil, cilantro, lime juice, lime zest, cumin, peppercorns, oregano, and salt.

2. Set in the refrigerator to marinate for 4 hours.

TO MAKE THE CHILI VERDE

1. Turn the oven broiler on high. Line an edged baking sheet with parchment paper.

2. Put the tomatillos, peppers, garlic, and onions onto the prepared baking sheet.

3. Broil for 5 minutes or until the vegetables start to blacken.

4. In a food processor, blend the vegetables, bone broth, cilantro, fennel, and salt for 1 minute or until smooth but still chunky.

5. Put the marinated pork into a 6-quart or larger slow cooker and cover with the chili.

6. Cover and cook on low for 6 hours or until the pork is fork-tender and falling apart.

7. Using two forks, shred the pork in the slow cooker, cool, and serve.

PER SERVING (1 CUP) CALORIES: 481; TOTAL FAT: 37G; SATURATED FAT: 11G; PROTEIN: 27G; TOTAL CARBOHYDRATES: 10G; FIBER: 3G; CHOLESTEROL: 107MG; MACROS: FAT: 69%; PROTEIN: 22%; CARBS: 9%

PORK PORTOBELLO PIZZA CAPS

ALLERGEN-FREE, EGG-FREE, NUT-FREE, QUICK PREP, UNDER 30 MINUTES

SERVES 4 | PREP TIME: **5 MINUTES** | COOK TIME: **20 MINUTES**

Enjoy subtle notes of all your favorite Italian pizza flavors in each delicious bite!

4 large portobello
  mushroom caps,
  wiped clean

2 tablespoons avocado
  oil, divided

Sea salt

Freshly ground black pepper

1 pound ground pork

2 medium garlic
  cloves, minced

2 cups tomato sauce

½ teaspoon Zesty Italian
  Seasoning (page 232)

1. Preheat the oven to 350°F. Line an edged baking sheet with parchment paper.

2. Brush the gill side of each mushroom cap with 1 tablespoon of avocado oil and season with salt and pepper.

3. Place the caps, gill-side up, on the prepared baking sheet.

4. Bake for 10 minutes or until the mushrooms are fork-tender.

5. Remove the mushrooms from the oven and set aside.

6. Heat the remaining 1 tablespoon of avocado oil in a large skillet over medium-high heat for 3 minutes or until the oil starts to shimmer.

7. Cook the pork and garlic for 5 minutes or until the pork is browned.

8. Carefully spoon one-quarter of the meat mixture into each mushroom cap.

9. In a small bowl, combine the tomato sauce and Italian seasoning and pour the sauce evenly over the mushroom caps.

10. Bake for 5 minutes or until the sauce is warm and fragrant. Serve immediately.

> **Variation Tip:** Top the pizza caps with toppings such as finely diced onions, bell peppers, or mushrooms before adding the sauce.

PER SERVING CALORIES: 351; TOTAL FAT: 23G; SATURATED FAT: 7G; PROTEIN: 24G; TOTAL CARBOHYDRATES: 12G; FIBER: 3G; CHOLESTEROL: 75MG; MACROS: FAT: 59%; PROTEIN: 27%; CARBS: 14%

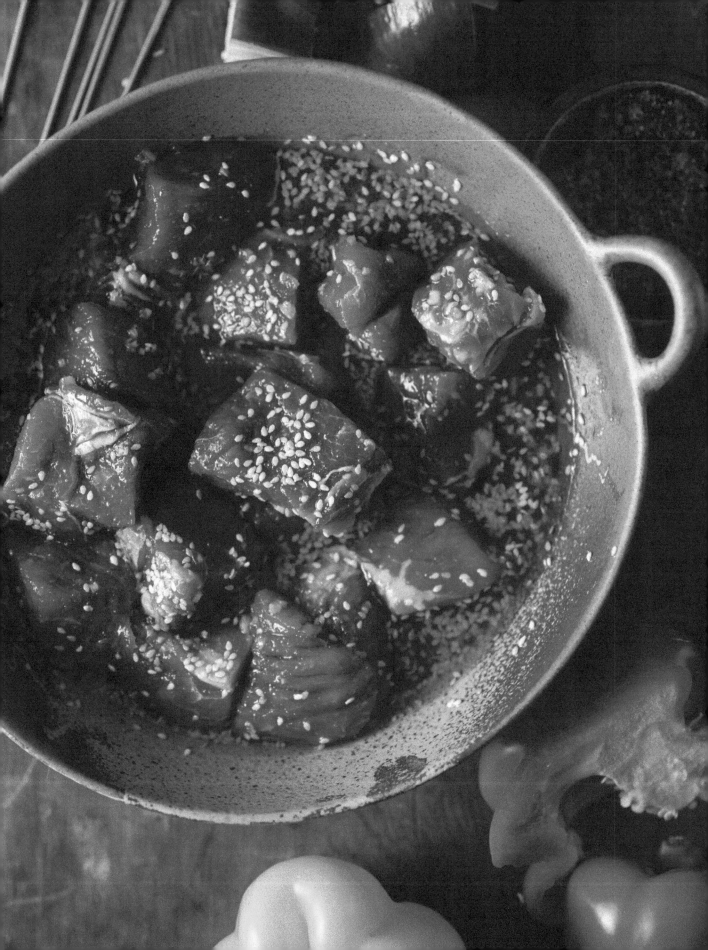

BEEF

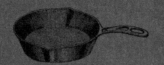

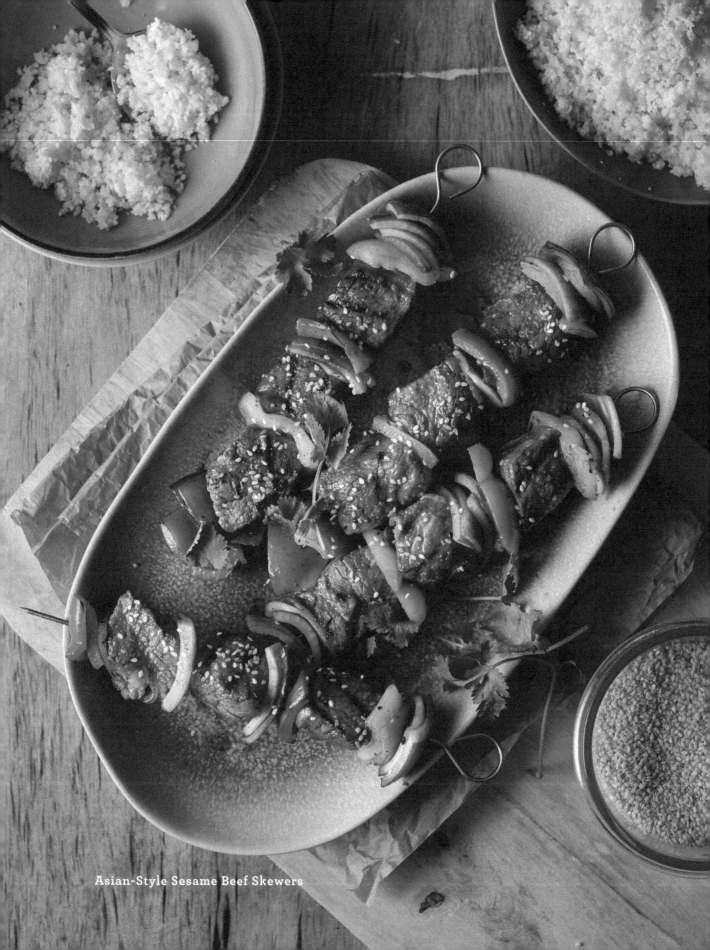

Asian-Style Sesame Beef Skewers

ASIAN-STYLE SESAME BEEF SKEWERS

ALLERGEN-FREE, EASY, EGG-FREE, NUT-FREE, QUICK PREP

SERVES 4 | PREP TIME: 10 MINUTES, PLUS 30 MINUTES TO MARINATE |
COOK TIME: **10 MINUTES**

Relish the sweet notes of coconut aminos and honey mixed with crunchy sesame seeds and minced ginger in each beefy bite.

1½ pounds rib eye steak, cut into 2-inch cubes

1 cup coconut aminos

½ cup extra-virgin olive oil, plus 1 tablespoon

1 tablespoon raw honey

2 tablespoons minced garlic

2 tablespoons sesame seeds

1 tablespoon minced peeled fresh ginger

1 teaspoon onion powder

½ teaspoon sea salt

1 large red onion, cut into 2-inch pieces

1 yellow bell pepper, cut into 2-inch pieces

1 red bell pepper, cut into 2-inch pieces

4 cups Grated Cauliflower Rice (page 37)

1. In a resealable quart-size bag, combine the steak, coconut aminos, ½ cup of olive oil, the honey, garlic, sesame seeds, ginger, onion powder, and salt.

2. Set in the refrigerator to marinate for 30 minutes. If using wooden skewers, start soaking them in water.

3. Heat the remaining 1 tablespoon of olive oil in a cast iron skillet over medium-high heat, or preheat a grill to medium-high heat (400°F).

4. Thread the skewers by alternating beef, bell pepper, and onion until all ingredients are used.

5. Place the skewers in the skillet or on the grill. Cook for 10 minutes, turning every 2 minutes to avoid burning, or until the beef is browned with an internal temperature of 145°F and the vegetables are soft.

6. Serve over a bed of cauliflower rice.

> **Variation Tip:** If fresh ginger is hard to find, you can use 1 teaspoon of ground ginger.

PER SERVING CALORIES: 618; TOTAL FAT: 46G; SATURATED FAT: 19G; PROTEIN: 34G; TOTAL CARBOHYDRATES: 17G; FIBER: 5G; CHOLESTEROL: 114MG; MACROS: FAT: 67%; PROTEIN: 22%; CARBS: 11%

TWO-MEATS LOAF

EASY, EGG-FREE

SERVES 8 | PREP TIME: **15 MINUTES** | COOK TIME: **1 HOUR 35 MINUTES**

This richly flavored meatloaf pairs well with Mashed Parsnips and Chives (page 198) or a side of steamed vegetables.

Coconut oil cooking spray

1 tablespoon extra-virgin olive oil

2 medium garlic cloves, minced

1 small white onion, finely chopped

2 small carrots, shredded

1 pound 80/20 ground beef

1 pound ground pork

½ cup blanched almond flour (page 29)

2 tablespoons tomato paste

1 tablespoon coconut aminos

1 tablespoon Dijon mustard

1 teaspoon freshly ground black pepper

1 teaspoon Zesty Italian Seasoning (page 232)

½ teaspoon sea salt

Sugar-Free Ketchup (page 235), for serving

1. Lightly grease a loaf pan with cooking spray. Set aside.

2. Preheat the oven to 350°F. Line an edged baking sheet with aluminum foil and top with an oven-safe wire rack covered with an additional piece of foil to keep the meatloaf from falling through the rack.

3. Heat the olive oil in a large skillet over medium-high heat for 3 minutes or until the oil starts to shimmer.

4. Sauté the garlic, onion, and carrots for 3 minutes or until the vegetables are soft. Transfer to a large bowl.

5. Add the beef, pork, almond flour, tomato paste, coconut aminos, mustard, pepper, Italian seasoning, and salt to the bowl with the vegetables. Combine.

6. Transfer the mixture to the prepared loaf pan. Using a spatula, spread the meatloaf so it is evenly distributed in the pan.

7. Turn the loaf pan upside down over the prepared baking sheet and allow the meatloaf to fall onto the wire rack. (If it doesn't come out easily, loosen the sides with a knife.)

8. Bake for 1 hour and 30 minutes or until the top has browned and the loaf is no longer pink in the middle.

9. Cool, slice, and serve with a dollop of home-made ketchup.

> **Ingredient Tip:** Make this dish allergen-free by swapping out the almond flour for 3 to 4 tablespoons of coconut flour.

PER SERVING CALORIES: 302; TOTAL FAT: 22G; SATURATED FAT: 7G; PROTEIN: 22G; TOTAL CARBOHYDRATES: 4G; FIBER: 1G; CHOLESTEROL: 67MG; MACROS: FAT: 66%; PROTEIN: 29%; CARBS: 5%

SLOPPY JOES

ALLERGEN-FREE, EASY, EGG-FREE, ONE-POT, QUICK PREP

SERVES 4 | PREP TIME: **10 MINUTES** | COOK TIME: **35 MINUTES**

Ditch the canned sloppy joe mix for this traditional homemade and healthy recipe!

1 tablespoon extra-virgin olive oil

1 medium white onion, chopped

1 medium bell pepper, chopped

2 medium garlic cloves, minced

1½ pounds 80/20 ground beef

1 cup tomato sauce

¼ cup coconut aminos

1 teaspoon apple cider vinegar

1 teaspoon chili powder

1 teaspoon ground paprika

½ teaspoon dried oregano

½ teaspoon cayenne powder

½ teaspoon sea salt

½ teaspoon freshly ground pepper

1. Heat the olive oil in a large skillet over medium-high heat for 3 minutes or until the oil starts to shimmer.

2. Sauté the onion, bell pepper, and garlic for 5 minutes or until the vegetables soften.

3. Add the ground beef and cook for an additional 5 minutes or until the meat is browned and no longer pink.

4. Add the tomato sauce, coconut aminos, apple cider vinegar, chili powder, paprika, oregano, cayenne, salt, and pepper. Stir to combine. Bring the contents to a boil, cover, and reduce the heat to low.

5. Simmer for 25 minutes or until the sauce has thickened and is fragrant.

Accompaniment Tip: Serve sloppy joes over paleo-approved tortilla chips or AIP/Allergen-Free Tortillas (page 36).

PER SERVING CALORIES: 485; TOTAL FAT: 33G; SATURATED FAT: 12G; PROTEIN: 34G; TOTAL CARBOHYDRATES: 13G; FIBER: 3G; CHOLESTEROL: 88MG; MACROS: FAT: 61%; PROTEIN: 28%; CARBS: 11%

SWEDISH MEATBALLS

SERVES 8 | PREP TIME: **15 MINUTES** | COOK TIME: **25 MINUTES**

Smothered in a rich, creamy gravy, these delicious Swedish meatballs are perfect for any dinner event or party.

FOR THE MEATBALLS

2 tablespoons coconut oil

1 pound 80/20 ground beef

1 pound ground pork

⅓ cup blanched almond flour (page 29)

1 large egg

½ medium white onion, finely chopped

2 tablespoons chopped fresh parsley

2 medium garlic cloves, minced

1 teaspoon sea salt

¼ teaspoon freshly ground black pepper

¼ teaspoon ground white pepper

⅛ teaspoon ground allspice

FOR THE GRAVY

3 tablespoons ghee

1½ tablespoons arrowroot flour

2 cups Beef Bone Broth (page 27)

½ cup full-fat coconut milk

1 teaspoon spicy brown mustard

1 tablespoon coconut aminos

Sea salt

Freshly ground black pepper

TO MAKE THE MEATBALLS

1. Heat the coconut oil in a large skillet over medium-high heat for 3 minutes or until the oil starts to shimmer.

2. In a large bowl, combine the beef, pork, almond flour, egg, onion, parsley, garlic, salt, black pepper, white pepper, and allspice. Roll the mixture into 24 (2-inch) meatballs.

3. Place the meatballs in an even layer in the skillet and cook in several batches, rotating the meatballs every 2 to 3 minutes to sear them evenly, until they are thoroughly browned.

4. Cook for an additional 5 minutes or until the meatballs are no longer pink in the middle and have an internal temperature of 165°F.

5. Using a slotted spoon, remove the meatballs and set aside. Pour out any remaining oil before returning the skillet to the burner.

TO MAKE THE GRAVY

1. Heat the ghee in the skillet over medium heat for 2 minutes or until it is melted.

2. Whisk in the arrowroot flour for 30 seconds or until it starts to bubble.

3. Slowly whisk in the bone broth, coconut milk, mustard, and coconut aminos. Season with salt and pepper.

4. Bring the gravy to a gentle boil. Using a slotted spoon, carefully place the meatballs back in the skillet and reduce the heat to low. Allow the gravy to thicken completely, about 3 to 5 minutes.

5. Use a slotted spoon to plate the meatballs and cover them with a generous amount of gravy. Serve immediately.

Variation Tip: Coconut milk can be swapped out for almond milk for a sweet and nuttier gravy.

PER SERVING CALORIES: 416; TOTAL FAT: 32G; SATURATED FAT: 16G; PROTEIN: 28G; TOTAL CARBOHYDRATES: 4G; FIBER: 1G; CHOLESTEROL: 102MG; MACROS: FAT: 69%; PROTEIN: 27%; CARBS: 4%

CHIMICHURRI PAN-SEARED RIB EYE

5 INGREDIENTS OR FEWER, ALLERGEN-FREE, EGG-FREE, NUT-FREE, ONE-POT, QUICK PREP, UNDER 30 MINUTES

SERVES 2 | PREP TIME: **5 MINUTES** | COOK TIME: **15 MINUTES**

Have dinner ready in under 30 minutes with these flavorful pan-seared steaks smothered in a delicious chimichurri sauce.

1 tablespoon avocado oil

2 (6-ounce) bone-in rib eye steaks, close to room temperature

Sea salt

Freshly ground black pepper

Chimichurri Sauce (page 241), for serving

1. Preheat the oven to 450°F.

2. Heat the avocado oil in a cast iron skillet over medium-high heat for 10 minutes or until the oil starts to shimmer.

3. Season the steaks with salt and pepper.

4. Sear the steaks for 5 minutes. Flip and sear for an additional 5 minutes or until they are crisp and brown.

5. Put the skillet directly into the preheated oven and cook for 5 minutes.

6. Transfer the steaks to a cutting board and allow them to rest for 5 minutes.

7. Slice the steak, drizzle with the chimichurri sauce, and serve.

> **Variation Tip:** Omit the chimichurri sauce for an AIP-friendly steak.

PER SERVING CALORIES: 500; TOTAL FAT: 44G; SATURATED FAT: 27G; PROTEIN: 25G; TOTAL CARBOHYDRATES: 1G; FIBER: 0G; CHOLESTEROL: 105MG; MACROS: FAT: 79%; PROTEIN: 20%; CARBS: 1%

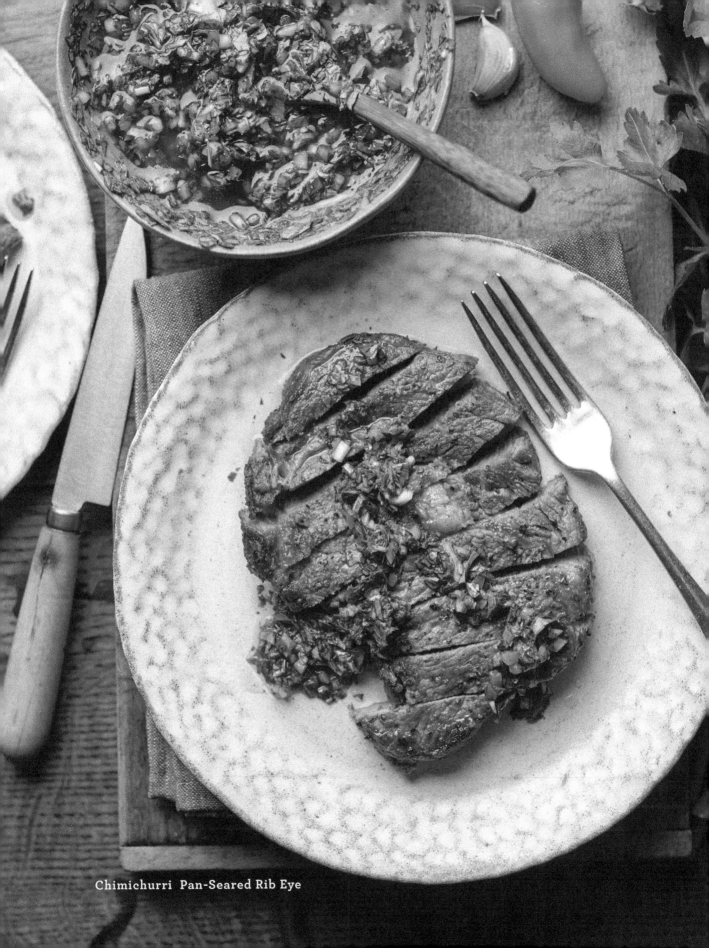

Chimichurri Pan-Seared Rib Eye

BEEF STROGANOFF

AIP-FRIENDLY, ALLERGEN-FREE, EASY, EGG-FREE, QUICK PREP

SERVES 4 | PREP TIME: **10 MINUTES** | COOK TIME: **6 HOURS**

Savor mouthwatering tender meat in a creamy, rich sauce that's loaded with mushrooms and served over a bed of mashed parsnips.

1½ pounds sirloin beef, cut into ⅛-inch-thick slices

½ teaspoon sea salt

½ teaspoon freshly ground black pepper

2 medium garlic cloves, minced

8 ounces cremini mushrooms, cut into ½-inch-thick slices

1¼ cups Beef Bone Broth (page 27)

½ cup full-fat coconut milk

¼ cup coconut aminos

3 tablespoons arrowroot flour

3 tablespoons water

Mashed Parsnips and Chives (page 198), for serving

1. Put the beef into a 6-quart or larger slow cooker. Season with the salt and pepper.

2. Top the beef with the garlic, mushrooms, bone broth, coconut milk, and coconut aminos.

3. Cover and cook on low for 6 hours or until the meat is fork-tender.

4. Thirty minutes before the meat is done, whisk together the arrowroot flour and water in a small bowl. Pour the mixture into the slow cooker, stir 3 or 4 times until the broth lightens, and cover. (The sauce will thicken as it sets.)

5. Serve over a bed of mashed parsnips.

> **Variation Tip:** Coconut milk can be swapped out for an equal amount of almond milk.

PER SERVING CALORIES: 449; TOTAL FAT: 17G; SATURATED FAT: 8G; PROTEIN: 50G; TOTAL CARBOHYDRATES: 24G; FIBER: 5G; CHOLESTEROL: 68MG; MACROS: FAT: 34%; PROTEIN: 45%; CARBS: 21%

BEEFY TACO CASSEROLE

SERVES 4 | PREP TIME: 10 MINUTES | COOK TIME: 40 MINUTES

Enjoy Mexican spices and tender vegetables married with homemade tortillas and fresh cilantro in this satisfying casserole.

Coconut oil cooking spray

1 tablespoon extra-virgin olive oil

¼ cup chopped white onion

¼ cup chopped bell pepper

2 medium garlic cloves, minced

1 pound 80/20 ground beef

2 tablespoons Two-Minute Taco Seasoning (page 231)

2 small zucchini, cut into ⅛-inch-thick slices

¼ cup black olives, drained and cut into ¼-inch-thick slices

¼ cup chopped frozen spinach

¼ cup chopped fresh cilantro

6 AIP/Allergen-Free Tortillas (page 36)

1 cup salsa, divided

1. Preheat the oven to 400°F. Lightly grease an 8-by-8-inch baking dish with cooking spray.

2. Heat the olive oil in a large skillet over medium-high heat for 3 minutes or until the oil starts to shimmer.

3. Sauté the onion, bell pepper, and garlic for 5 minutes or until the vegetables soften.

4. Add the ground beef and cook for 5 minutes or until the meat is no longer pink. Season the beef and vegetables with the taco seasoning.

5. Add the zucchini, olives, spinach, and cilantro. Cover and cook for an additional 8 minutes or until the zucchini is fork-tender and the spinach is warmed through.

6. To assemble the casserole, layer the bottom of the prepared dish with tortillas, tearing the tortillas as needed to cover the bottom. Top with half the ground beef and vegetables and ½ cup of salsa. Repeat this step one additional time.

7. Bake for 20 minutes or until the top is brown. Serve immediately.

> **Variation Tip:** Try making chicken taco casserole by swapping out the beef for shredded chicken.

PER SERVING CALORIES: 435; TOTAL FAT: 27G; SATURATED FAT: 11G; PROTEIN: 24G; TOTAL CARBOHYDRATES: 24G; FIBER: 5G; CHOLESTEROL: 59MG; MACROS: FAT: 56%; PROTEIN: 22%; CARBS: 22%

SLOW-COOKER BEEF ROAST WITH GRAVY

ALLERGEN-FREE, EASY, EGG-FREE, NUT-FREE, QUICK PREP

SERVES 6 | PREP TIME: 10 MINUTES | COOK TIME: **6 HOURS**

Come home and warm up with this delicious, perfectly seasoned, tender chuck roast with hearty vegetables.

2½ pounds bone-in chuck roast

1 teaspoon garlic powder

1 teaspoon onion powder

1 teaspoon ground paprika

1 teaspoon chili powder

1 teaspoon sea salt

1 teaspoon freshly ground black pepper

2 large white onions, quartered

3 medium carrots, cut into ¼-inch-thick slices

2 small sweet potatoes, peeled and cut into 1-inch chunks

2 tablespoons arrowroot flour

2 tablespoons water

1. Put the chuck roast into a 6-quart or larger slow cooker.

2. In a small bowl, combine the garlic powder, onion powder, paprika, chili powder, salt, and pepper. Sprinkle half of the seasoning over the roast.

3. Add the onions, carrots, and sweet potatoes to the slow cooker and sprinkle with the remaining seasoning.

4. Cover and cook on low for 6 hours or until the vegetables are tender and the meat is falling off the bone.

5. Carefully remove the roast and vegetables and discard the bone. Leave the meat juices in the slow cooker to make a gravy.

6. In a small bowl, whisk together the arrowroot flour and water. Add the mixture to the slow cooker and stir 3 or 4 times until the sauce lightens. The sauce will thicken as it sets.

7. Return the meat and vegetables to the slow cooker and cover with the gravy. Allow to rest for 5 minutes and serve.

> Variation Tip: Swap out or add your favorite vegetables to this roast. Asparagus, mushrooms, parsnips, and butternut squash are just a few of the options that work well.

PER SERVING CALORIES: 439; TOTAL FAT: 27G; SATURATED FAT: 11G; PROTEIN: 33G; TOTAL CARBOHYDRATES: 16G; FIBER: 4G; CHOLESTEROL: 112MG; MACROS: FAT: 55%; PROTEIN: 30%; CARBS: 15%

GAME DAY CHILI

SERVES 6 | PREP TIME: **10 MINUTES** | COOK TIME: **6 HOURS**

Everyone loves a game day chili, especially the cook!

FOR THE CHILI SEASONING

1 tablespoon chili powder

1 teaspoon ground cumin

1 teaspoon ground coriander

1 teaspoon ground paprika

1 teaspoon dried oregano

1 teaspoon garlic powder

1 teaspoon onion powder

1 teaspoon sea salt

1 teaspoon freshly ground
   black pepper

FOR THE CHILI

1 pound 80/20 ground beef

1 (14-ounce) can
   diced tomatoes

1 (14-ounce) can
   tomato sauce

1 (6-ounce) can
   tomato paste

2 medium carrots, cut into
   ¼-inch-thick slices

1 medium sweet potato,
   peeled and cut into
   ½-inch chunks

1 medium white
   onion, chopped

1 bell pepper, chopped

TO MAKE THE CHILI SEASONING

In a small bowl, combine the chili powder, cumin, coriander, paprika, oregano, garlic powder, onion powder, salt, and pepper. Set aside.

TO MAKE THE CHILI

1. In a 6-quart or larger slow cooker, combine the beef, diced tomatoes with their juices, tomato sauce, tomato paste, carrots, sweet potato, onion, and bell pepper.

2. Sprinkle in the chili seasoning, cover, and cook for 6 hours on low or until the vegetables are tender and the beef is no longer pink. Serve immediately.

Variation Tip: Swap out ground beef for ground pork or chicken.

PER SERVING CALORIES: 290; TOTAL FAT: 14G; SATURATED FAT: 5G; PROTEIN: 18G; TOTAL CARBOHYDRATES: 23G; FIBER: 6G; CHOLESTEROL: 39MG; MACROS: FAT: 43%; PROTEIN: 25%; CARBS: 32%

LASAGNA

EGG-FREE

SERVES 6 | PREP TIME: **25 MINUTES** | COOK TIME: **35 MINUTES**

This delicious, nutrient-packed meal lets you enjoy the traditional flavors of lasagna without the grain and dairy.

FOR THE CASHEW CHEESE

2 cups raw cashews

½ cup warm water

¼ cup nutritional yeast

2 tablespoons freshly squeezed lemon juice

2 teaspoons Zesty Italian Seasoning (page 232)

1 teaspoon sea salt

FOR THE LASAGNA

1 pound 80/20 ground beef

1 pound ground pork

1 large white onion, chopped

2 garlic cloves, minced

4 cups Garden-Fresh Spaghetti Sauce (page 240)

2 cups chopped baby spinach

6 medium zucchini, cut into ⅛-inch-thick slices

TO MAKE THE CASHEW CHEESE

In a food processor, blend the cashews, water, nutritional yeast, lemon juice, Italian seasoning, and salt for 1 to 2 minutes or until smooth and creamy with no visible cashew chunks. Set aside.

TO MAKE THE LASAGNA

1. Sauté the ground beef, pork, onion, and garlic in a large skillet over medium-high heat for 5 minutes or until the beef and pork are no longer pink.

2. Add the spaghetti sauce and spinach and stir for 30 seconds or until the spinach is wilted. Remove from the heat.

3. Preheat the oven to 350°F.

4. To assemble the lasagna, layer the bottom of a 9-by-13-inch baking dish with zucchini slices.

5. With a spatula, spread a single layer of cashew cheese on top of the zucchini slices, then top with one-third of the meat sauce. Repeat until all the ingredients are used (roughly 3 layers).

6. Cook the lasagna uncovered for 30 minutes or until the sides start to bubble up and the top starts to brown. Allow to set for 5 minutes before serving.

> **Prep Tip:** It may be easier to assemble your lasagna by cutting the zucchini slices in half.

PER SERVING CALORIES: 788; TOTAL FAT: 52G; SATURATED FAT: 14G; PROTEIN: 46G; TOTAL CARBOHYDRATES: 34G; FIBER: 8G; CHOLESTEROL: 89MG; MACROS: FAT: 59%; PROTEIN: 23%; CARBS: 18%

BEEF AND BROCCOLI STIR-FRY

ALLERGEN-FREE, EGG-FREE, QUICK PREP

SERVES 4 | PREP TIME: 10 MINUTES | COOK TIME: 20 MINUTES

Enjoy tender beef and vegetables covered in a delicious sauce made from sweet coconut aminos and honey combined with freshly grated ginger.

---

2 tablespoons extra-virgin olive oil, divided

1½ pounds precut sirloin beef strips

2 medium garlic cloves, minced

½ teaspoon sea salt

½ teaspoon freshly ground black pepper

⅓ cup coconut aminos

1 tablespoon raw honey

1 tablespoon peeled grated fresh ginger

1 tablespoon arrowroot flour

1 tablespoon warm water

1 large white onion, cut into ¼-inch-thick slices

1 medium head broccoli, cut into ½-inch florets

1 bell pepper, cut into ¼-inch-thick slices

4 ounces cremini mushrooms, cut into ¼-inch-thick slices

4 cups Grated Cauliflower Rice (page 37)

1. Heat 1 tablespoon of olive oil in a large skillet over medium-high heat for 3 minutes or until the oil starts to shimmer.

2. Sauté the beef strips and garlic with salt and pepper for 3 minutes or until the beef is brown (do not overcook).

3. In a small saucepan, combine the coconut aminos, honey, and ginger over medium heat.

4. In a small bowl, whisk together the arrowroot flour and water for 20 seconds or until smooth. Pour the mixture into the small saucepan with the coconut aminos mixture and stir for 30 seconds or until the sauce starts to thicken. Remove from the heat.

5. Transfer the cooked meat from the skillet to the saucepan. Return the skillet to the burner. Heat the remaining 1 tablespoon of olive oil over medium-high heat for 3 minutes or until the oil starts to shimmer.

6. Sauté the onion, broccoli, bell pepper, and mushrooms for 5 minutes or until the onion is translucent.

7. Add the beef with sauce, cover, and reduce the heat to medium-low. Cook for an additional 10 minutes or until the broccoli is fork-tender. Serve over a bed of cauliflower rice.

Prep Tip: This recipe is a great grab-and-go option. Store in individual airtight containers in the refrigerator for up to 3 days.

PER SERVING CALORIES: 383; TOTAL FAT: 11G; SATURATED FAT: 1G; PROTEIN: 45G; TOTAL CARBOHYDRATES: 26G; FIBER: 7G; CHOLESTEROL: 89MG; MACROS: FAT: 26%; PROTEIN: 47%; CARBS: 27%

CORNED BEEF AND CABBAGE

AIP-FRIENDLY, ALLERGEN-FREE, EASY, EGG-FREE, NUT-FREE

SERVES 6 | PREP TIME: 15 MINUTES, PLUS 48 HOURS TO MARINATE | COOK TIME: 8 HOURS

For tender, flavorful corned beef, it's best to cure it yourself with a water-based brine and whole mustard seeds and peppercorns. I promise the results are worth the wait!

FOR THE BRINE

3 pounds brisket

4 cups warm water, more if needed

½ cup fine sea salt

1 tablespoon whole mustard seeds

1 tablespoon ground mustard

1 tablespoon whole black peppercorns

1 teaspoon ground ginger

1 teaspoon whole cloves

FOR THE CORNED BEEF AND CABBAGE

4 cups Beef Bone Broth (page 27)

4 cups shredded cabbage

4 medium carrots, cut into ¼-inch-thick slices

1 large white onion, cut into ½-inch-thick slices

1 tablespoon whole mustard seeds

1 teaspoon whole black peppercorns

2 bay leaves

TO MAKE THE BRINE

1. Put the brisket in a 2-quart container or one that is large enough to hold the brisket and brine.

2. In a medium bowl, combine the warm water and salt until the salt dissolves. Pour the water over the brisket until it is fully immersed (add more water as needed). If the brisket starts floating, weigh it down with a plate.

3. Add the mustard seeds, ground mustard, peppercorns, ginger, and cloves.

4. Cover and set in the refrigerator for 48 hours.

5. After 48 hours, remove the brisket, rinse, and transfer to a 6-quart or larger slow cooker.

TO MAKE THE CORNED BEEF AND CABBAGE

1. To the brisket, add the bone broth, cabbage, carrots, onion, mustard seeds, peppercorns, and bay leaves.

2. Cook on low for 8 hours or until the brisket is falling apart and the carrots are fork-tender.

3. Remove the brisket from the slow cooker and shred or carve into ⅛-inch-thick slices.

4. Serve immediately with the cabbage and carrots.

> **Ingredient Tip:** Since it is not cured with pink curing salt (sodium nitrate), the beef will not have a pink hue.

PER SERVING CALORIES: 399; TOTAL FAT: 15G; SATURATED FAT: 1G; PROTEIN: 53G; TOTAL CARBOHYDRATES: 13G; FIBER: 4G; CHOLESTEROL: 76MG; MACROS: FAT: 34%; PROTEIN: 52%; CARBS: 14%

PRIME RIB AND HORSERADISH SAUCE

EASY, NUT-FREE

SERVES 4 | PREP TIME: **15 MINUTES** | COOK TIME: **55 MINUTES**

Enjoy restaurant-quality, oven-roasted prime rib topped with a tangy and creamy home-made horseradish sauce without leaving the house.

FOR THE HORSERADISH SAUCE

1 cup Real Paleo Mayonnaise (page 234)

½ cup peeled chopped horseradish root

1 medium garlic clove, minced

FOR THE PRIME RIB

3 pounds standing rib roast

Sea salt

Freshly ground black pepper

TO MAKE THE HORSERADISH SAUCE

In a food processor, blend the mayonnaise, horseradish, and garlic on high for 1 minute or until smooth and creamy.

TO MAKE THE PRIME RIB

1. Preheat the oven to 450°F.

2. Season all sides of the roast generously with salt and pepper and put it in a roasting pan.

3. Roast for 20 minutes, then reduce the temperature to 325°F and roast for an additional 35 minutes or until the internal temperature reaches 130°F for medium-rare.

4. Transfer the roast to a cutting board and allow it to rest for 20 minutes.

5. Cut the roast into ¼-inch-thick slices and serve with a dollop of horseradish sauce.

Prep Tip: For well-done meat, aim for an internal temperature of 145°F.

PER SERVING CALORIES: 545; TOTAL FAT: 49G; SATURATED FAT: 18G; PROTEIN: 26G; TOTAL CARBOHYDRATES: 0G; FIBER: 0G; CHOLESTEROL: 106MG; MACROS: FAT: 80%; PROTEIN: 19%; CARBS: 1%

BRAISED BEEF SHORT RIBS

ALLERGEN-FREE, EASY, EGG-FREE, NUT-FREE

SERVES 4 | PREP TIME: **20 MINUTES** | COOK TIME: **3 HOURS 10 MINUTES**

These short ribs are slow cooked for a fall-off-the-bone finish.

---

4 bone-in short ribs

Sea salt

Freshly ground black pepper

¼ cup arrowroot flour

6 nitrate- and sugar-free bacon slices, chopped

3 tablespoons avocado oil

6 medium garlic cloves, minced

1 large white onion, chopped

3 medium carrots, peeled and chopped

2 medium celery stalks, chopped

2 cups red wine

2 cups Beef Bone Broth (page 27)

2 thyme sprigs

2 rosemary sprigs

1. Preheat the oven to 325°F.

2. Generously season the short ribs with salt and pepper.

3. Pour the arrowroot flour into a small bowl. Dredge each short rib in the flour to coat each side. Set the ribs aside.

4. Sauté the bacon in a Dutch oven or oven-proof stock-pot over medium-high heat for 5 minutes, stirring until the bacon is cooked and browned.

5. With a slotted spoon, remove the bacon and place it onto a paper towel–lined plate to remove the excess grease. Set aside.

6. Add the avocado oil to the bacon drippings and sear the ribs by rotating every minute until all sides are browned. Remove the short ribs and set aside.

7. In the same pot, sauté the garlic, onion, carrots, and celery for 2 minutes or until the onion softens.

8. Add the red wine and deglaze the bottom of the pot, gently scraping and stirring up the browned bits from the bottom. Bring to a boil.

9. Add the beef broth, thyme, rosemary, short ribs, and bacon bits and cover. Put the pot into the oven and bake for 3 hours or until the ribs are fork-tender.

10. Allow the ribs to rest on the stovetop for 20 minutes before serving.

PER SERVING CALORIES: 573; TOTAL FAT: 41G; SATURATED FAT: 14G; PROTEIN: 35G; TOTAL CARBOHYDRATES: 16G; FIBER: 2G; CHOLESTEROL: 121MG; MACROS: FAT: 64%; PROTEIN: 24%; CARBS: 12%

SLOW-COOKED BEEF BRISKET

AIP-FRIENDLY, ALLERGEN-FREE, EASY, EGG-FREE, NUT-FREE

SERVES 4 TO 6 | PREP TIME: 15 MINUTES | COOK TIME: 8 HOURS 10 MINUTES

If you don't have time to make Mashed Parsnips and Chives or Mushroom Gravy, this brisket tastes amazing topped with my favorite homemade Date-Infused Barbecue Sauce (page 237).

1 tablespoon extra-virgin olive oil

3 pounds beef brisket

1 teaspoon sea salt

1 teaspoon freshly ground black pepper

1 large white onion, cut into ½-inch-thick slices

4 large garlic cloves, peeled

2 bay leaves

½ cup Beef Bone Broth (page 27)

Mashed Parsnips and Chives (page 198), for serving

Mushroom Gravy (page 239), for serving

1. Heat the olive oil in a cast iron skillet over medium-high heat for 3 minutes or until the oil starts to shimmer.

2. Season the brisket with salt and pepper.

3. Sear the seasoned brisket for 3 minutes. Flip and sear for an additional 3 minutes or until both sides are crisp and browned.

4. Transfer the brisket to a 6-quart or larger slow cooker and top with the onion, garlic, bay leaves, and bone broth. Cover and cook on low for 8 hours or until the brisket is fork-tender.

5. Remove the brisket from the slow cooker and cut into ¼-inch-thick slices.

6. Serve over a bed of mashed parsnips and top with mushroom gravy.

> **Make-Ahead Tip:** Prepare your brisket and side dishes the night before for a quick weeknight meal.

PER SERVING (6 OUNCES) CALORIES: 651; TOTAL FAT: 47G; SATURATED FAT: 19G; PROTEIN: 37G; TOTAL CARBOHYDRATES: 20G; FIBER: 4G; CHOLESTEROL: 135MG; MACROS: FAT: 65%; PROTEIN: 23%; CARBS: 12%

GRILLED SKIRT STEAK FAJITAS

ALLERGEN-FREE, EASY, EGG-FREE, QUICK PREP

SERVES 4 | PREP TIME: 10 MINUTES, PLUS 2 HOURS TO MARINATE | COOK TIME: 20 MINUTES

Enjoy the sweetness of the coconut aminos, the heat from the chili powder and red pepper flakes, and the freshness of cilantro in these zesty fajitas.

2 pounds skirt steak

½ cup avocado oil, plus 1 tablespoon

3 tablespoons coconut aminos

¼ cup freshly squeezed lime juice

4 medium garlic cloves, minced

1 tablespoon chopped fresh cilantro

1 tablespoon ground cumin

1 tablespoon chili powder

1 tablespoon coconut sugar

½ teaspoon red pepper flakes

1 teaspoon sea salt

½ teaspoon freshly ground black pepper

1 large white onion, cut into ¼-inch-thick slices

1 red bell pepper, cut into ¼-inch-thick slices

1 orange bell pepper, cut into ¼-inch-thick slices

1 yellow bell pepper, cut into ¼-inch-thick slices

4 AIP/Allergen-Free Tortillas (page 36)

1. In a resealable quart-size bag, combine the skirt steak, ½ cup of avocado oil, the coconut aminos, lime juice, garlic, cilantro, cumin, chili powder, coconut sugar, red pepper flakes, salt, and pepper.

2. Let the steak marinate in the refrigerator for 2 hours.

3. Meanwhile, heat the remaining 1 tablespoon of avocado oil in a large skillet over medium-high heat for 3 minutes or until the oil starts to shimmer.

4. Sauté the onion and bell peppers for 8 minutes or until the vegetables are soft and the onion is translucent. Remove the vegetables from the skillet and set aside.

5. Heat the skillet over medium-high heat, or preheat a grill to medium-high heat (400°F).

6. Remove the marinated skirt steak from the bag and cook it in the skillet or on the grill for 4 minutes. Flip and cook for an additional 4 minutes or until the steak has a crisp, brown finish.

7. Transfer the skirt steak to a cutting board and allow it to rest for 10 minutes before cutting into ⅛-inch-thick slices.

8. Serve over the tortillas and top with the sautéed onion and bell peppers.

Variation Tip: Skirt steak can be swapped out for flank steak; both will yield tender results.

PER SERVING CALORIES: 681; TOTAL FAT: 37G; SATURATED FAT: 14G; PROTEIN: 63G; TOTAL CARBOHYDRATES: 24G; FIBER: 4G; CHOLESTEROL: 162MG; MACROS: FAT: 49%; PROTEIN: 37%; CARBS: 14%

SPICY BEEF AND SWEET POTATOES

ALLERGEN-FREE, EASY, EGG-FREE, NUT-FREE, ONE-POT, QUICK PREP

SERVES 4 | PREP TIME: 10 MINUTES | COOK TIME: 20 MINUTES

Spice up the night with this warming beef and sweet potato dish. If you're not a huge fan of spicy foods, cut back the jalapeño or omit it completely.

1 tablespoon extra-virgin olive oil

½ medium white onion, chopped

½ jalapeño, chopped

2 medium garlic cloves, minced

1 pound 80/20 ground beef

½ teaspoon sea salt

½ teaspoon freshly ground black pepper

½ teaspoon ground paprika

⅛ teaspoon ground nutmeg

2 cups sweet potatoes, cut into ½-inch chunks

1. Heat the olive oil in a large skillet over medium-high heat for 3 minutes or until the oil starts to shimmer.

2. Sauté the onion, jalapeño, and garlic for 5 minutes or until the onion begins to brown.

3. Add the ground beef, salt, pepper, paprika, and nutmeg and cook for 5 minutes or until the meat is no longer pink.

4. Add the sweet potato, cover, and reduce the heat to medium. Cook for 10 minutes or until the potatoes are fork-tender.

Variation Tip: Replace the ground beef with ground pork or shredded chicken.

PER SERVING CALORIES: 363; TOTAL FAT: 23G; SATURATED FAT: 8G; PROTEIN: 23G; TOTAL CARBOHYDRATES: 16G; FIBER: 3G; CHOLESTEROL: 59MG; MACROS: FAT: 57%; PROTEIN: 26%; CARBS: 17%

ROASTED PORTOBELLO MUSHROOM BURGERS

AIP-FRIENDLY, ALLERGEN-FREE, EASY, EGG-FREE, NUT-FREE, QUICK PREP

SERVES 4 | PREP TIME: **10 MINUTES** | COOK TIME: **25 MINUTES**

Ditch the grain burger buns for these fun and delicious roasted portobello mushroom caps!

FOR THE MUSHROOM BUNS

8 large portobello mushroom caps, wiped clean

2 tablespoons extra-virgin olive oil

Sea salt

Freshly ground black pepper

FOR THE BURGERS

1 tablespoon extra-virgin olive oil

1 pound 80/20 ground beef

1 teaspoon sea salt

1 teaspoon freshly ground black pepper

1 teaspoon dried oregano

1 teaspoon garlic powder

1 teaspoon onion powder

TO MAKE THE MUSHROOM BUNS

1. Preheat the oven to 450°F. Line a baking sheet with parchment paper.

2. Brush the gill side of the mushrooms with the olive oil and season with salt and pepper. Place the caps, gill-side up, on the prepared baking sheet. Roast for 10 to 12 minutes or until the mushrooms are fork-tender. Remove from the oven and set aside.

TO MAKE THE BURGERS

1. Heat the olive oil in a cast iron skillet over medium-high heat for 3 minutes or until the oil starts to shimmer.

2. Divide the ground beef into 4 equal pieces and roll into balls. Flatten each ball between two pieces of parchment paper or foil to form round, 1-inch-thick burgers.

3. In a small bowl, combine the salt, pepper, oregano, garlic powder, and onion powder. Season both sides of each burger.

4. Cook the beef patties for 5 minutes or until brown. Flip the patties, cover, and cook for an additional 5 minutes or until the internal temperature is 150°F for a medium-well burger. Remove the burgers from the skillet and let them rest for 5 minutes before serving.

5. Sandwich each burger between mushroom caps, top with your favorite burger toppings, and serve.

PER SERVING CALORIES: 414; TOTAL FAT: 30G; SATURATED FAT: 9G; PROTEIN: 26G; TOTAL CARBOHYDRATES: 10G; FIBER: 3G; CHOLESTEROL: 59MG; MACROS: FAT: 65%; PROTEIN: 25%; CARBS: 10%

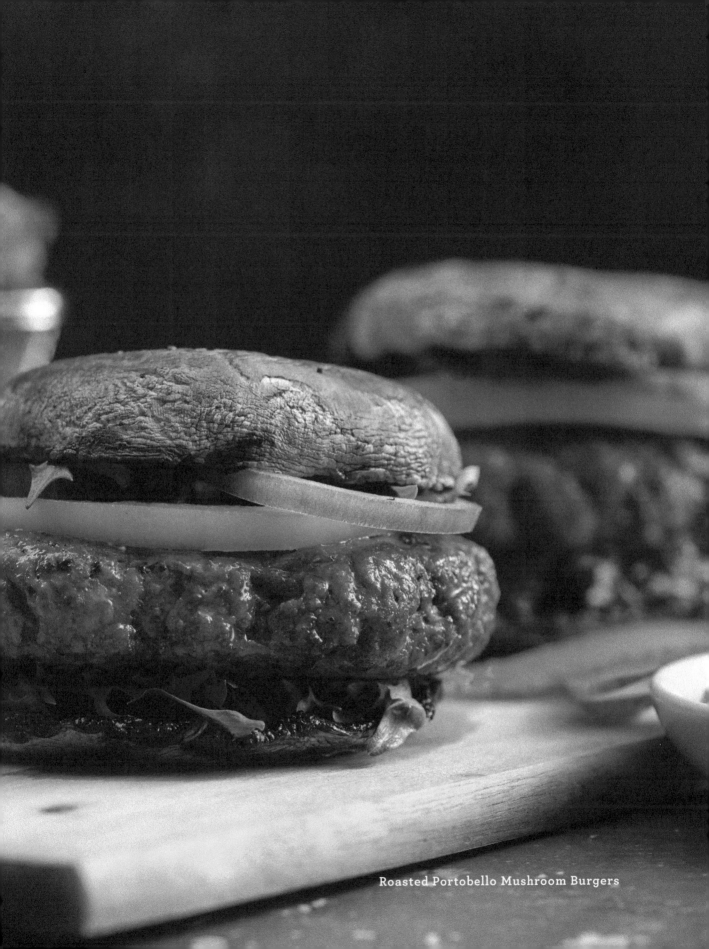

Roasted Portobello Mushroom Burgers

ZESTY ITALIAN BEEF

5 INGREDIENTS OR FEWER, ALLERGEN-FREE, EASY, EGG-FREE, NUT-FREE, QUICK PREP

SERVES 4 TO 6 | PREP TIME: **5 MINUTES** | COOK TIME: **6 HOURS**

This zesty Italian beef is marinated in beef broth and the pepperoncini liquid and seasoned to perfection.

---

3 pounds beef chuck roast

1 large white onion, cut into ½-inch-thick slices

1 (12-ounce) jar pepperoncini, plus liquid

2 cups Beef Bone Broth (page 27)

1 tablespoon Zesty Italian Seasoning (page 232)

1. Put the chuck roast into a 6-quart or larger slow cooker and top with the onion, pepperoncini and their liquid, bone broth, and Italian seasoning.

2. Cover and cook on low for 6 hours or until the meat is fork-tender.

3. Transfer the roast to a cutting board and let cool before shredding with a fork.

4. Return the meat to the slow cooker and immerse it in the broth before serving.

> **Make-Ahead Tip:** To reduce the cooking time by several hours, first freeze the roast for 2 hours beforehand, then cut it into thin slices before cooking.

PER SERVING (6 OUNCES) CALORIES: 459; TOTAL FAT: 27G; SATURATED FAT: 10G; PROTEIN: 45G; TOTAL CARBOHYDRATES: 9G; FIBER: 1G; CHOLESTEROL: 133MG; MACROS: FAT: 53%; PROTEIN: 39%; CARBS: 8%

ITALIAN MEATBALLS

EASY, QUICK PREP

SERVES 4 | PREP TIME: 5 MINUTES | COOK TIME: 30 MINUTES
Combining ground beef, pork, and fresh seasonings, these meatballs make a fantastic appetizer or a tasty main dish!

½ pound 80/20 ground beef

½ pound ground pork

½ small white onion, chopped

2 medium garlic cloves, minced

1 large egg

2 tablespoons blanched almond flour (page 29)

2 tablespoons chopped fresh parsley

½ teaspoon sea salt

1 teaspoon freshly ground black pepper

1. Preheat the oven to 350°F. Line a baking sheet with aluminum foil and top with an oven-safe wire rack.

2. In a large bowl, combine the ground beef, pork, onion, garlic, egg, almond flour, parsley, salt, and pepper.

3. Roll the mixture into 1½-inch balls and place the meatballs on the prepared wire rack in a single layer.

4. Cook for 30 minutes or until the meatballs are cooked through and no longer pink in the middle.

5. Allow the meatballs to cool on the rack for 5 minutes before serving.

Variation Tip: Turn your meatballs into a classic-inspired dish by making Zucchini Noodles (Zoodles, page 32) and Garden-Fresh Spaghetti Sauce (page 240).

PER SERVING CALORIES: 280; TOTAL FAT: 20G; SATURATED FAT: 7G; PROTEIN: 23G; TOTAL CARBOHYDRATES: 2G; FIBER: 1G; CHOLESTEROL: 113MG; MACROS: FAT: 64%; PROTEIN: 33%; CARBS: 3%

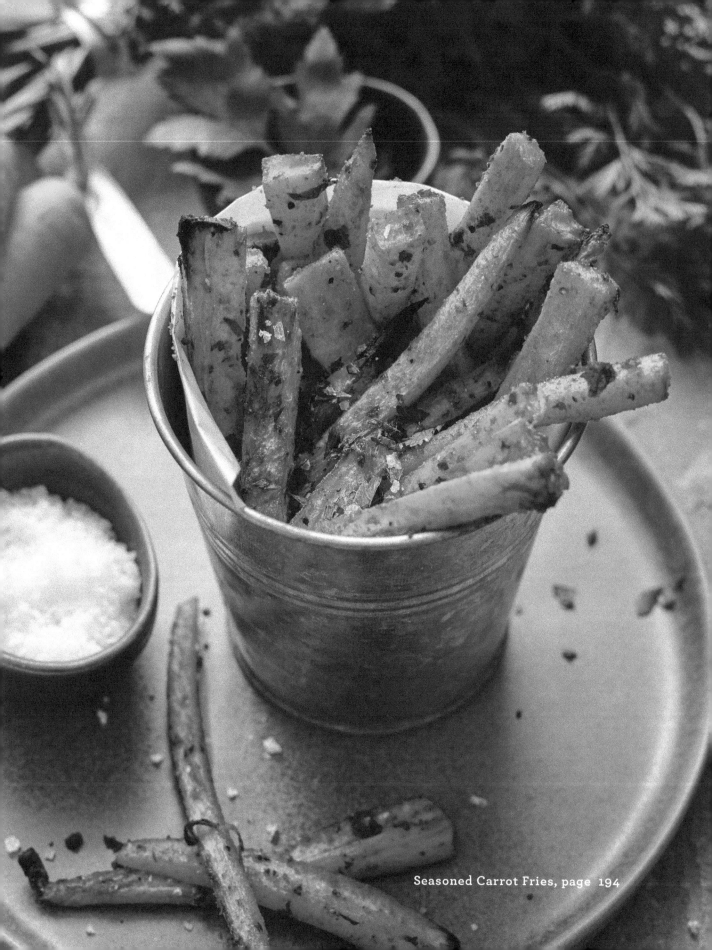

Seasoned Carrot Fries, page 194

SNACKS AND SIDES

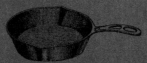

SEASONED CARROT FRIES

SERVES 2 TO 4 | PREP TIME: **10 MINUTES** | COOK TIME: **20 MINUTES**

These perfectly seasoned carrot fries are baked in the oven until they are tender on the inside with a beautiful outer crisp!

6 large carrots,
   peeled and cut into
   ⅛-inch-thick slices

2 tablespoons extra-virgin
   olive oil

1 tablespoon chopped
   fresh parsley

1 teaspoon ground paprika

1 teaspoon ground cumin

½ teaspoon sea salt

1 teaspoon freshly ground
   black pepper

1. Preheat the oven to 425°F. Line an edged baking sheet with parchment paper.

2. In a large bowl, combine the carrots, olive oil, parsley, paprika, cumin, salt, and pepper.

3. Arrange the carrots in a single layer on the baking sheet.

4. Bake for 20 minutes or until the carrots are slightly crispy. Serve immediately.

Variation Tip: If you don't have fresh parsley on hand, you can use dried parsley or fresh or dried oregano. Adjust dried spices accordingly.

PER SERVING (½ CUP) CALORIES: 226; TOTAL FAT: 14G; SATURATED FAT: 2G; PROTEIN: 2G; TOTAL CARBOHYDRATES: 23G; FIBER: 6G; CHOLESTEROL: 0MG; MACROS: FAT: 56%; PROTEIN: 3%; CARBS: 41%

HASSELBACK SWEET POTATOES

5 INGREDIENTS OR FEWER, AIP-FRIENDLY, ALLERGEN-FREE, EGG-FREE, NUT-FREE, QUICK PREP

SERVES 4 | PREP TIME: **10 MINUTES** | COOK TIME: **45 MINUTES**

These Hasselback sweet potatoes are cut two-thirds of the way through to create thin slices that are topped with extra-virgin olive oil and garlic and seasoned with salt and pepper.

2 large sweet potatoes,
skins on

4 tablespoons extra-virgin
olive oil, divided

2 garlic cloves,
minced, divided

1 teaspoon sea salt, divided

1 teaspoon freshly ground
black pepper, divided

1. Preheat the oven to 425°F. Line an edged baking sheet with parchment paper.

2. Make a series of ⅛-inch slices along each sweet potato, slicing only two-thirds of the way through, and place onto the prepared baking sheet.

3. Brush 2 tablespoons of olive oil over the first sweet potato, working to get the oil in between all the slices.

4. Add half of the minced garlic, ½ teaspoon of salt, and ½ teaspoon of pepper.

5. Repeat steps 3 and 4 for the other sweet potato.

6. Bake for 45 minutes or until the center is fork-tender and the outside is crisp. Cool before serving.

> **Variation Tip:** Make Hasselback sweet potatoes on the grill by following steps 2 through 5, then wrapping the potatoes tightly in aluminum foil. Cook on medium-high (400°F) away from direct heat for 45 minutes or until fork-tender.

PER SERVING CALORIES: 185; TOTAL FAT: 14G; SATURATED FAT: 2G; PROTEIN: 1G; TOTAL CARBOHYDRATES: 14G; FIBER: 2G; CHOLESTEROL: 0MG; MACROS: FAT: 68%; PROTEIN: 2%; CARBS: 30%

BACON-ROASTED BRUSSELS SPROUTS

5 INGREDIENTS OR FEWER, AIP-FRIENDLY, ALLERGEN-FREE, EASY, EGG-FREE, NUT-FREE, QUICK PREP

SERVES 4 | PREP TIME: **10 MINUTES** | COOK TIME: **35 MINUTES**

Some say it's possible, but in my mind, you can't eat Brussels sprouts without the bacon!

1 pound nitrate- and sugar-free bacon

1 pound Brussels sprouts, quartered

Sea salt

Freshly ground black pepper

1. Preheat the oven to 425°F. Line an edged baking sheet with aluminum foil.

2. Place the bacon on the prepared baking sheet (the slices should overlap as little as possible). Bake for 13 minutes or until brown and crispy.

3. Remove the bacon from the baking sheet, reserving the drippings, and put them on a paper towel–lined plate to remove excess grease. Crumble the bacon into bits and set aside.

4. In a large bowl, combine the Brussels sprouts and bacon drippings until each Brussels sprout is evenly coated. Season with salt and pepper.

5. Put the Brussels sprouts on the same baking sheet and bake for 20 minutes or until they are crisp and fork-tender. Top with the bacon and serve.

Variation Tip: The bacon can be cooked in a skillet over medium-high heat for 5 minutes per side or until brown and crispy. Save the drippings!

PER SERVING CALORIES: 521; TOTAL FAT: 45G; SATURATED FAT: 15G; PROTEIN: 18G; TOTAL CARBOHYDRATES: 12G; FIBER: 4G; CHOLESTEROL: 77MG; MACROS: FAT: 78%; PROTEIN: 14%; CARBS: 8%

CINNAMON SUGAR APPLESAUCE

5 INGREDIENTS OR FEWER, AIP-FRIENDLY, ALLERGEN-FREE, EGG-FREE, QUICK PREP

MAKES 8 CUPS | PREP TIME: **10 MINUTES** | COOK TIME: **30 MINUTES**

Bring all the warm autumnal flavors together in this homemade cinnamon sugar apple-sauce. I love using sweeter apples (like Gala), but you can use whatever apples you have on hand.

8 apples, peeled, cored, and cut into ¼-inch-thick slices

1 cup water

¼ cup coconut sugar

1 teaspoon cinnamon

1. In a large stockpot, combine the apples, water, coconut sugar, and cinnamon over medium heat for 10 minutes or until boiling.

2. Cover and reduce the heat to low. Simmer for 20 minutes or until the apples break apart with a fork.

3. Remove the stockpot from the burner and cool.

4. Transfer the contents to a food processor and blend for 1 minute or until smooth with no visible apple chunks. Serve or refrigerate immediately.

> **Variation Tip:** Coconut sugar can be replaced with raw honey or omitted entirely for a sugar-free option.

PER SERVING (½ CUP) CALORIES: 52; TOTAL FAT: 0G; SATURATED FAT: 0G; PROTEIN: 0G; TOTAL CARBOHYDRATES: 13G; FIBER: 1G; CHOLESTEROL: 0MG; MACROS: FAT: 0%; PROTEIN: 1%; CARBS: 99%

MASHED PARSNIPS AND CHIVES

SERVES 2 TO 4 | PREP TIME: **10 MINUTES** | COOK TIME: **20 MINUTES**

Pair this side dish with Beef Stroganoff (page 176) or Slow-Cooked Beef Brisket (page 185) to make any meal into a comfort meal.

2 large parsnips, peeled and cut into 1-inch chunks

¼ cup full-fat coconut milk, more if needed

1 tablespoon chopped fresh chives

¼ teaspoon sea salt

¼ teaspoon freshly ground black pepper

1. Fill a medium stockpot halfway with water and bring it to a boil.

2. Carefully put the parsnips into the pot with a slotted spoon and boil for 20 minutes or until fork-tender.

3. Drain the parsnips and transfer them to a large bowl.

4. Add the coconut milk, chives, salt, and pepper.

5. Using a potato masher or fork, mash the parsnips for 1 minute or until smooth. If the mixture is too thick, add extra coconut milk, 1 tablespoon at a time, until the parsnips are smooth and creamy. Serve immediately.

> **Variation Tip:** Coconut milk can be swapped out for almond milk.

PER SERVING (½ CUP) CALORIES: 184; TOTAL FAT: 8G; SATURATED FAT: 6G; PROTEIN: 3G; TOTAL CARBOHYDRATES: 26G; FIBER: 7G; CHOLESTEROL: 0MG; MACROS: FAT: 39%; PROTEIN: 4%; CARBS: 57%

CLASSIC SWEET POTATO CASSEROLE

EASY, EGG-FREE

SERVES 8 | PREP TIME: **15 MINUTES** | COOK TIME: **1 HOUR**

Turn your traditional casserole dish into a healthy version that even your old-school grandmother will love.

FOR THE SWEET POTATO MASH

4 medium sweet potatoes, peeled and cut into 1-inch chunks

¼ cup full-fat coconut milk, more if needed

1 teaspoon sea salt

1 teaspoon freshly ground black pepper

FOR THE PECAN TOPPING

1 cup roughly chopped pecans

3 tablespoons pure maple syrup

2 tablespoons melted grass-fed butter or coconut oil

½ teaspoon vanilla extract

½ teaspoon ground cinnamon

⅛ teaspoon sea salt

TO MAKE THE SWEET POTATO MASH

1. In a medium stockpot, cover the sweet potatoes with water. Bring to a boil over medium-high heat. Boil for 20 minutes or until fork-tender.

2. Drain the sweet potatoes and allow them to cool.

3. In a food processor, blend the sweet potatoes, coconut milk, salt, and pepper on high for 1 minute or until smooth and creamy. (If the mixture is too thick, add extra coconut milk, 1 tablespoon at a time, until it is smooth and creamy.)

4. Pour into an 8-by-8-inch edged baking dish and smooth down with a spatula.

TO MAKE THE PECAN TOPPING

1. Preheat the oven to 375°F.

2. In a medium bowl, combine the pecans, maple syrup, butter, vanilla, cinnamon, and salt. Pour the mixture evenly over the sweet potatoes.

3. Cover with aluminum foil and bake for 20 minutes.

4. Remove the foil and bake for an additional 20 minutes or until the pecans are browned and glazed. Cool and serve.

Variation Tip: Swap out the pecans for walnuts or almonds to change up this sweet potato casserole, or use tigernuts for an AIP-friendly and allergen-free dish.

PER SERVING CALORIES: 249; TOTAL FAT: 17G; SATURATED FAT: 6G; PROTEIN: 3G; TOTAL CARBOHYDRATES: 21G; FIBER: 4G; CHOLESTEROL: 0MG; MACROS: FAT: 61%; PROTEIN: 5%; CARBS: 34%

BALSAMIC BROCCOLI AND MUSHROOM SKILLET

ALLERGEN-FREE, EASY, EGG-FREE, UNDER 30 MINUTES

SERVES 4 | PREP TIME: **15 MINUTES** | COOK TIME: **10 MINUTES**

This one-pan, veggie-packed skillet is perfect for a quick side dish, and it pairs well with just about any protein.

1 medium head broccoli, cut into 1-inch florets

1 tablespoon extra-virgin olive oil

8 ounces cremini mushrooms, cut into ¼-inch-thick slices

2 medium garlic cloves, minced

2 tablespoons balsamic vinegar

1 tablespoon coconut aminos

¼ teaspoon sea salt

¼ teaspoon red pepper flakes

1. Fill a medium stockpot halfway with water and bring to a boil over medium-high heat.

2. Using a slotted spoon, add the broccoli florets into the pot and boil for 3 minutes or until fork-tender. Drain the broccoli and set aside.

3. Heat the olive oil in a large skillet over medium-high heat for 3 minutes or until the oil starts to shimmer.

4. Sauté the mushrooms and garlic for 5 minutes or until the mushrooms are browned.

5. Remove the skillet from the heat and add the balsamic vinegar, coconut aminos, salt, red pepper flakes, and broccoli. Gently toss and serve.

> **Variation Tip:** Cremini mushrooms can be swapped out for shiitake mushrooms or any other mushrooms you like.

PER SERVING CALORIES: 96; TOTAL FAT: 4G; SATURATED FAT: 1G; PROTEIN: 5G; TOTAL CARBOHYDRATES: 11G; FIBER: 3G; CHOLESTEROL: 0MG; MACROS: FAT: 38%; PROTEIN: 16%; CARBS: 46%

GRAIN-FREE VANILLA AND MAPLE GRANOLA

EASY, EGG-FREE, QUICK PREP, UNDER 30 MINUTES

MAKES 3 CUPS | PREP TIME: **5 MINUTES** | COOK TIME: **15 MINUTES**

This granola is sweetened with pure maple syrup and seasoned with cinnamon and salt, making it the perfect sweet and salty treat.

1½ cups unsweetened coconut flakes

¾ cup sliced almonds

¾ cup chopped pecans

½ cup sunflower seeds

1 teaspoon ground cinnamon

½ teaspoon sea salt

4 tablespoons pure maple syrup

1 tablespoon melted coconut oil

1 teaspoon vanilla extract

1. Preheat the oven to 300°F. Line an edged baking sheet with parchment paper.

2. In a large bowl, combine the coconut flakes, almonds, pecans, sunflower seeds, cinnamon, and salt.

3. In a small bowl, whisk together the maple syrup, coconut oil, and vanilla.

4. Pour the syrup mixture over the nuts and seeds and stir until they are evenly coated.

5. Using a spatula, spread the mixture onto the prepared baking sheet as evenly as possible and bake for 15 minutes or until the almonds and coconut flakes are golden brown.

6. Cool completely on the baking sheet before serving or storing.

Storage Tip: The granola will stay fresh in an airtight container or resealable bag for 5 days.

PER SERVING (3 TABLESPOONS) CALORIES: 161; TOTAL FAT: 13G; SATURATED FAT: 6G; PROTEIN: 3G; TOTAL CARBOHYDRATES: 8G; FIBER: 3G; CHOLESTEROL: 0MG; MACROS: FAT: 73%; PROTEIN: 7%; CARBS: 20%

MAPLE ACORN SQUASH

5 INGREDIENTS OR FEWER, AIP-FRIENDLY, ALLERGEN-FREE, EGG-FREE, NUT-FREE, QUICK PREP

SERVES 2 | PREP TIME: **10 MINUTES** | COOK TIME: **1 HOUR**

This maple acorn squash pairs well with many of the pork recipes in this book, especially the Pan-Seared Pork Chops (page 151).

---

1 small acorn squash, halved lengthwise

2 tablespoons extra-virgin olive oil

2 tablespoons pure maple syrup

¼ teaspoon sea salt

½ teaspoon freshly ground black pepper

1. Preheat the oven to 400°F. Line an edged baking sheet with parchment paper.

2. Put the acorn squash, cut-side up, on the prepared baking sheet.

3. In a small bowl, whisk together the olive oil, maple syrup, salt, and pepper.

4. Generously brush the yellow rims of the acorn squash with the mixture and pour half of the rest of the mixture into each half of the squash.

5. Bake for 60 minutes or until the squash is fork-tender and easily shreds away from its skin. Cool and serve.

> Variation Tip: Maple syrup can be replaced with coconut sugar. Just be sure to heat the mixture and stir to dissolve the sugar before using.

PER SERVING CALORIES: 278; TOTAL FAT: 14G; SATURATED FAT: 2G; PROTEIN: 2G; TOTAL CARBOHYDRATES: 36G; FIBER: 3G; CHOLESTEROL: 0MG; MACROS: FAT: 45%; PROTEIN: 3%; CARBS: 52%

NITRATE-FREE BEEF JERKY

ALLERGEN-FREE, EASY, EGG-FREE, QUICK PREP

MAKES 24 STRIPS | PREP TIME: 10 MINUTES, PLUS 24 HOURS TO MARINATE |
COOK TIME: **4 HOURS**

This jerky is perfect for on-the-go snacks, hiking, and camping trips. Enjoy the subtle hints of spice from the chipotle and paprika powder toned down with the sweetness of the coconut aminos.

1½ pounds flank steak, cut into 1/10-inch-thick slices

2 garlic cloves, minced

½ cup coconut aminos

1 teaspoon chipotle powder

1 teaspoon ground paprika

1 teaspoon onion powder

1 teaspoon garlic powder

1 teaspoon sea salt

1 teaspoon freshly ground black pepper

1. In a resealable quart-size bag, combine the steak, garlic, coconut aminos, chipotle powder, paprika, onion powder, garlic powder, salt, and pepper.

2. Set the steak in the refrigerator to marinate for 24 hours.

3. Preheat the oven to 170°F. Line an edged baking sheet with aluminum foil and top with an oven-safe wire rack.

4. Lay the strips of meat onto the prepared wire rack in a single layer. Cook for 3 to 4 hours or until the meat has a dark brown (not burnt) outer layer but is still tender.

5. Allow to cool completely. Serve or store.

> **Storage Tip:** Store jerky in an airtight container in a cool, dark place for 2 weeks or in the refrigerator for 1 month.

PER SERVING (4 STRIPS) CALORIES: 210; TOTAL FAT: 10G; SATURATED FAT: 0G; PROTEIN: 25G; TOTAL CARBOHYDRATES: 5G; FIBER: 0G; CHOLESTEROL: 0MG; MACROS: FAT: 43%; PROTEIN: 48%; CARBS: 9%

NATURE'S TRAIL MIX

MAKES 8 CUPS | PREP TIME: **5 MINUTES**

Enjoy this sweet and salty mix full of nutrient-dense fats and proteins. Store extra trail mix in an airtight container for up to 3 months.

---

8 ounces whole raw cashews

8 ounces whole raw almonds

8 ounces raw pistachios, shelled

1 cup paleo chocolate chips or chunks

1. In a large bowl, combine the cashews, almonds, pistachios, and chocolate.

2. Serve immediately or store in an airtight container.

> **Variation Tip:** Sweeten your trail mix with raisins instead of chocolate and add a tart note with unsweetened dried cranberries.

PER SERVING (¼ CUP) CALORIES: 183; TOTAL FAT: 15G; SATURATED FAT: 4G; PROTEIN: 5G; TOTAL CARBOHYDRATES: 7G; FIBER: 4G; CHOLESTEROL: 0MG; MACROS: FAT: 74%; PROTEIN: 11%; CARBS: 15%

CLASSIC DEVILED EGGS

EASY, NUT-FREE, QUICK PREP, UNDER 30 MINUTES

MAKES 12 EGGS | PREP TIME: **10 MINUTES**

It's not a real party until the deviled eggs make an appearance.

6 hard-boiled eggs, peeled and halved lengthwise

¼ cup Real Paleo Mayonnaise (page 234)

1 teaspoon yellow mustard

1 teaspoon white vinegar

⅛ teaspoon sea salt

¼ teaspoon freshly ground black pepper

Ground paprika, for sprinkling

1. Gently remove the yolks from the eggs and put them into a small mixing bowl. Arrange the white halves on an egg platter or serving dish.

2. Mash the yolks with a fork until finely crumbled. Fold in the mayonnaise, mustard, white vinegar, salt, and pepper. Stir until smooth and creamy.

3. Using a piping bag, spoon, or a plastic bag with a corner cut off, fill each egg half with 1 to 1½ tablespoons of the yolk mixture. Sprinkle with paprika.

4. Serve immediately.

Variation Tip: Make the eggs ahead of time by baking them in the oven! Place 1 egg into each cup of a muffin tin and bake in the oven at 350°F for 30 minutes. Immerse the eggs in an ice bath for 10 minutes before peeling or storing.

PER SERVING (1 EGG) CALORIES: 66; TOTAL FAT: 6G; SATURATED FAT: 2G; PROTEIN: 3G; TOTAL CARBOHYDRATES: 0G; FIBER: 0G; CHOLESTEROL: 86MG; MACROS: FAT: 82%; PROTEIN: 16%; CARBS: 2%

BACON-WRAPPED ASPARAGUS

5 INGREDIENTS OR FEWER, AIP-FRIENDLY, ALLERGEN-FREE, EGG-FREE, NUT-FREE, QUICK PREP

SERVES 4 | PREP TIME: **5 MINUTES** | COOK TIME: **25 MINUTES**

Turn any dull party into a fun one with this two-ingredient appetizer.

12 medium asparagus spears, trimmed

12 nitrate- and sugar-free bacon slices

1. Preheat the oven to 425°F. Line an edged baking sheet with aluminum foil and top with an oven-safe wire rack.

2. Wrap each asparagus spear with bacon and place onto the prepared wire rack in a single layer.

3. Bake for 20 minutes or until the bacon is brown and slightly crisp.

4. Turn the broiler on high for 3 to 5 minutes. Flip the asparagus with tongs halfway through for all-around crispy bacon.

5. Serve immediately.

Make-Ahead Tip: Whip up a quick spicy aioli dipping sauce by combining ⅓ cup of Real Paleo Mayonnaise (page 234), ½ teaspoon of cayenne powder, and 2 minced garlic cloves.

PER SERVING CALORIES: 316; TOTAL FAT: 24G; SATURATED FAT: 8G; PROTEIN: 22G; TOTAL CARBOHYDRATES: 3G; FIBER: 1G; CHOLESTEROL: 63MG; MACROS: FAT: 68%; PROTEIN: 28%; CARBS: 4%

LOADED TWICE-BAKED SWEET POTATOES

ALLERGEN-FREE, EASY, EGG-FREE, NUT-FREE

SERVES 6 | PREP TIME: **15 MINUTES** | COOK TIME: **1 HOUR 15 MINUTES**

These potatoes are the perfect substitution for traditional twice-baked white potatoes thanks to their lower glycemic index and sweet flavor.

---

3 medium sweet potatoes, skin on

3 tablespoons full-fat coconut milk

1 tablespoon nutritional yeast

1 teaspoon spicy brown mustard

¼ teaspoon sea salt

¼ teaspoon freshly ground black pepper

3 scallions, white and green parts, chopped

6 nitrate- and sugar-free bacon slices, cooked and crumbled

1 jalapeño, chopped (optional)

1. Preheat the oven to 400°F. Line an edged baking sheet with parchment paper.

2. Pierce the sweet potatoes all over with a fork. Put the potatoes on the prepared baking sheet and bake for 1 hour or until fork-tender. Remove from the oven and let cool.

3. Cut the sweet potatoes in half lengthwise. Scoop out the flesh into a medium bowl while leaving the skin intact.

4. In a food processor, blend the sweet potato flesh, coconut milk, nutritional yeast, mustard, salt, and pepper on high for 1 minute or until smooth and creamy.

5. Fold in the scallions, bacon, and jalapeño (if using).

6. Return the mixture to the sweet potato skins and bake for 15 minutes or until the tops are crispy. Serve immediately.

> **Variation Tip:** Coconut milk can be replaced with almond milk.

PER SERVING CALORIES: 195; TOTAL FAT: 10G; SATURATED FAT: 4G; PROTEIN: 10G; TOTAL CARBOHYDRATES: 16G; FIBER: 3G; CHOLESTEROL: 21MG; MACROS: FAT: 46%; PROTEIN: 21%; CARBS: 33%

ROASTED CAULIFLOWER AND RED PEPPER HUMMUS

ALLERGEN-FREE, EASY, EGG-FREE, NUT-FREE, QUICK PREP

SERVES 8 | PREP TIME: **10 MINUTES** | COOK TIME: **20 MINUTES**

This appetizer is not only paleo but also allergen-free and vegan, making it satisfying and versatile for all guests.

---

1 medium head cauliflower, cut into 1-inch florets

½ red bell pepper, cut into ½-inch-thick slices

4 tablespoons extra-virgin olive oil, divided

½ teaspoon sea salt

½ teaspoon freshly ground black pepper

½ cup tahini

4 garlic cloves, minced

1 tablespoon freshly squeezed lemon juice

1 teaspoon ground cumin

1. Preheat the oven to 425°F. Line an edged baking sheet with parchment paper.

2. In a large bowl, combine the cauliflower, bell pepper, 1 tablespoon of olive oil, the salt, and pepper.

3. Arrange the vegetables on the prepared baking sheet and bake for 20 minutes or until the cauliflower is fork-tender. Remove from the oven and let cool.

4. In a food processor, blend the vegetables, the remaining 3 tablespoons of olive oil, the tahini, garlic, lemon juice, and cumin on high for 1 minute or until smooth and creamy. Serve immediately or store in an airtight container for up to 3 days in the refrigerator.

Ingredient Tip: If the hummus is too thick, add extra olive oil, a tablespoon at a time, until it has the desired consistency.

PER SERVING CALORIES: 248; TOTAL FAT: 20G; SATURATED FAT: 3G; PROTEIN: 6G; TOTAL CARBOHYDRATES: 11G; FIBER: 5G; CHOLESTEROL: OMG; MACROS: FAT: 73%; PROTEIN: 9%; CARBS: 18%

ROASTED HONEY-MUSTARD SWEET POTATO SALAD

ALLERGEN-FREE, EASY, EGG-FREE, NUT-FREE

SERVES 8 | PREP TIME: 15 MINUTES | COOK TIME: **35 MINUTES**

This side dish is perfect for summer barbecues and pairs excellent with my Dry-Rubbed Ribs (page 145).

FOR THE HONEY MUSTARD DRESSING

2 tablespoons raw honey

2 tablespoons Dijon mustard

2 tablespoons freshly squeezed lemon juice

½ teaspoon sea salt

½ teaspoon freshly ground black pepper

FOR THE SWEET POTATO SALAD

2 large sweet potatoes, peeled and cut into 1-inch chunks

2 tablespoons extra-virgin olive oil

1 teaspoon sea salt

1 teaspoon freshly ground black pepper

3 scallions, white and green parts, chopped

2 medium celery stalks, chopped

1 red bell pepper, chopped

TO MAKE THE HONEY MUSTARD DRESSING

In a small bowl, whisk together the honey, mustard, lemon juice, salt, and pepper until smooth and creamy. Set aside.

TO MAKE THE SWEET POTATO SALAD

1. Preheat the oven to 400°F. Line an edged baking sheet with parchment paper.

2. In a large bowl, combine the sweet potatoes, olive oil, salt, and pepper.

3. Arrange the potatoes on the prepared baking sheet in a single layer and bake for 35 to 40 minutes or until fork-tender. Remove from the oven and let cool.

4. In the large bowl, combine the sweet potatoes, scallions, celery, bell pepper, and honey mustard dressing, stirring until the vegetables are evenly coated. Best if served cold.

Make-Ahead Tip: Make this dish up to 24 hours in advance and store in the refrigerator in an airtight container.

PER SERVING CALORIES: 92; TOTAL FAT: 4G; SATURATED FAT: 1G; PROTEIN: 1G; TOTAL CARBOHYDRATES: 13G; FIBER: 2G; CHOLESTEROL: 0MG; MACROS: FAT: 39%; PROTEIN: 4%; CARBS: 57%

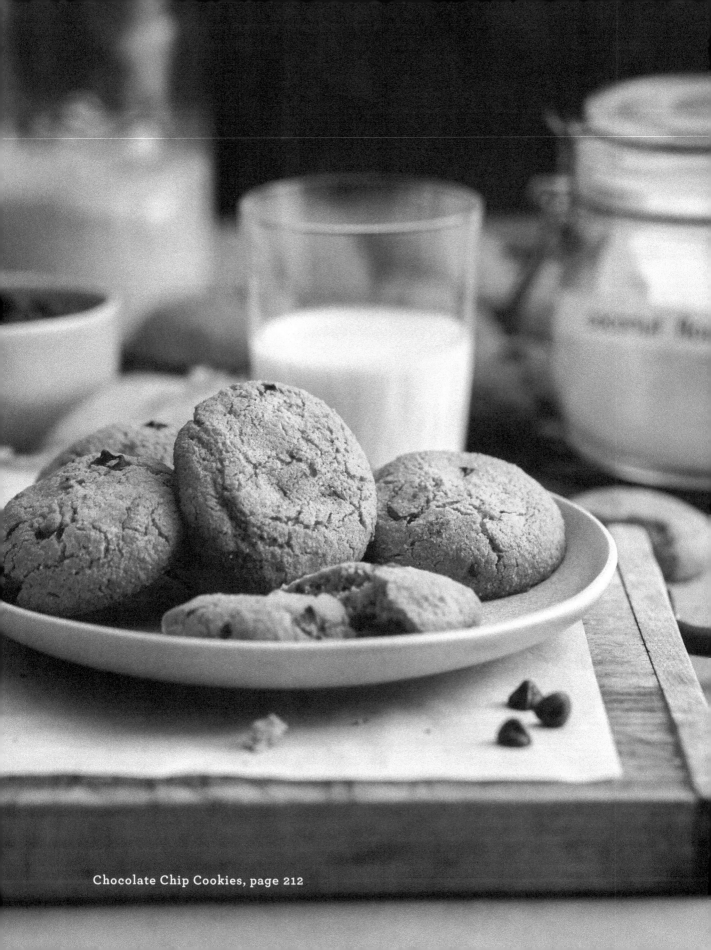

Chocolate Chip Cookies, page 212

SWEETS

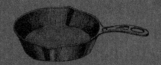

CHOCOLATE CHIP COOKIES

EASY, QUICK PREP, UNDER 30 MINUTES

MAKES 24 COOKIES | PREP TIME: **10 MINUTES** | COOK TIME: **10 MINUTES**

Nothing takes me back to my childhood quicker than the smell of burnt chocolate chip cookies. Though my mom wasn't the greatest cook, she did try. I hope you will try these moist and chewy (and not burnt!) chocolate chip cookies.

¾ cup coconut sugar

½ cup coconut oil

1 large egg,
   room temperature

1 teaspoon vanilla extract

1 cup arrowroot flour

½ cup coconut flour

½ teaspoon baking soda

½ teaspoon sea salt

1 cup paleo chocolate chips
   or chunks

1. Preheat the oven to 350°F. Line an edged baking sheet with parchment paper.

2. In a large bowl, beat the coconut sugar and oil until smooth. Add the egg and vanilla.

3. In a medium bowl, combine the arrowroot flour, coconut flour, baking soda, and salt.

4. Slowly add the dry ingredients to the wet ingredients and mix well until evenly combined.

5. Fold in the chocolate chips and spoon the dough onto the prepared baking sheet.

6. Bake for 10 minutes or until the cookies are golden brown. Cool on the baking sheet before serving.

Ingredient Tip: Make homemade chocolate chips by combining ¾ cup of coconut oil, ¾ cup of cacao powder, ⅓ cup of maple syrup, and 1 teaspoon of vanilla extract in a small saucepan over medium heat until melted. Pour the chocolate into a chocolate chip silicone mold and harden in the refrigerator.

PER SERVING (1 COOKIE) CALORIES: 163; TOTAL FAT: 11G; SATURATED FAT: 8G; PROTEIN: 3G; TOTAL CARBOHYDRATES: 13G; FIBER: 3G; CHOLESTEROL: 8MG; MACROS: FAT: 61%; PROTEIN: 7%; CARBS: 32%

MAPLE PECANS

SERVES 8 | PREP TIME: **5 MINUTES** | COOK TIME: **20 MINUTES**

These pecans are baked and naturally sweetened with maple syrup for a sweet and crunchy treat. Enjoy a few or a handful!

---

1 pound raw pecans, halved

¼ cup pure maple syrup

Sea salt

1. Preheat the oven to 325°F. Line a 12-by-17-inch edged baking sheet with parchment paper.

2. In a large bowl, combine the pecans and maple syrup until the pecans are evenly coated.

3. Pour the pecans onto the prepared baking sheet in a single layer and bake for 10 minutes. Stir with a wooden spoon.

4. Bake for an additional 10 minutes or until the pecans have a shiny glaze.

5. Remove from the oven, season with salt, and cool.

> **Storage Tip:** Store in an airtight container for up to 2 weeks.

PER SERVING CALORIES: 453; TOTAL FAT: 41G; SATURATED FAT: 4G; PROTEIN: 6G; TOTAL CARBOHYDRATES: 15G; FIBER: 6G; CHOLESTEROL: 0MG; MACROS: FAT: 81%; PROTEIN: 6%; CARBS: 13%

HONEY GLAZED CASHEWS

SERVES 8 | PREP TIME: **5 MINUTES** | COOK TIME: **10 MINUTES**

Ditch the store-bought honey cashews and their unnecessary additives and sugars for this simple and delicious homemade alternative.

---

1 pound whole raw cashews

1 tablespoon raw honey

Sea salt

2 tablespoons coconut sugar

1. Preheat the oven to 350°F. Line a 12-by-17-inch edged baking sheet with parchment paper.

2. In a large bowl, combine the cashews and honey until the cashews are evenly coated.

3. Pour the cashews onto the prepared baking sheet in a single layer, season with sea salt, and bake for 5 minutes. Stir with a wooden spoon.

4. Bake for an additional 5 minutes or until the cashews are a light golden brown.

5. Sprinkle the coconut sugar onto the cashews immediately and stir with a wooden spoon until they are evenly coated. Cool before serving.

> **Storage Tip:** Store in an airtight container for up to 2 weeks.

PER SERVING CALORIES: 354; TOTAL FAT: 26G; SATURATED FAT: 4G; PROTEIN: 10G; TOTAL CARBOHYDRATES: 20G; FIBER: 6G; CHOLESTEROL: 0MG; MACROS: FAT: 66%; PROTEIN: 11%; CARBS: 23%

ALMOND BUTTER–FILLED CHOCOLATE CUPS

5 INGREDIENTS OR FEWER, EASY, EGG-FREE, QUICK PREP

MAKES 24 CHOCOLATE CUPS | PREP TIME: 10 MINUTES, PLUS 30 MINUTES TO SET | COOK TIME: 5 MINUTES

These are the perfect treat for parties, holidays, or anytime you need an almond butter and chocolate fix.

---

1 cup paleo chocolate chips or chunks

½ cup almond butter

⅓ cup coconut flour

4 tablespoons pure maple syrup

1. Line the cups of a mini-muffin tin with liners.

2. In a small saucepan, melt the chocolate over low heat for 5 minutes or until completely melted, stirring occasionally to avoid burning the chocolate.

3. In a medium bowl, combine the almond butter, coconut flour, and maple syrup.

4. Roll the almond butter mixture into 24 balls.

5. Pour ½ teaspoon of melted chocolate into the bottom of each muffin cup and top with one ball. Press down slightly.

6. Cover each of the balls with an additional ½ teaspoon of melted chocolate or more to cover completely.

7. Set the pan in the freezer for 30 minutes or until the cups have hardened. Serve immediately or keep in the refrigerator for up to 5 days.

> Variation Tip: Swap out the almond butter for sunflower butter to make this an allergen-free treat.

PER SERVING (1 CHOCOLATE CUP) CALORIES: 90; TOTAL FAT: 6G; SATURATED FAT: 4G; PROTEIN: 2G; TOTAL CARBOHYDRATES: 7G; FIBER: 3G; CHOLESTEROL: 0MG; MACROS: FAT: 60%; PROTEIN: 9%; CARBS: 31%

CINNAMON ROLL MUG CAKE

SERVES 1 | PREP TIME: 5 MINUTES | COOK TIME: 2 MINUTES

This cinnamon roll mug cake is the closest thing you will get to the real deal in under 10 minutes.

¼ cup paleo pancake and waffle mix

1 tablespoon coconut sugar

¼ teaspoon ground cinnamon

¼ teaspoon baking powder

2 tablespoons almond milk

1 tablespoon pure maple syrup

1 teaspoon coconut oil

¼ teaspoon vanilla extract

1. In an 8-ounce or larger coffee mug, combine the pancake mix, coconut sugar, cinnamon, and baking powder.

2. Whisk in the almond milk, maple syrup, coconut oil, and vanilla until evenly combined.

3. Microwave for 1 minute and 30 seconds or until the cake has risen and the top is golden brown.

4. Carefully remove from the microwave and cool before serving.

Accompaniment Tip: Add a sweet cream glaze by whisking together ¼ cup of coconut cream and 2 tablespoons of pure maple syrup.

PER SERVING CALORIES: 240; TOTAL FAT: 8G; SATURATED FAT: 6G; PROTEIN: 4G; TOTAL CARBOHYDRATES: 38G; FIBER: 3G; CHOLESTEROL: 50MG; MACROS: FAT: 30%; PROTEIN: 7%; CARBS: 63%

BLONDIE BROWNIES

EASY, QUICK PREP

MAKES 12 BROWNIES | PREP TIME: 10 MINUTES | COOK TIME: **20 MINUTES**

These blondie brownies are so good, you'll forget they are free of grains, dairy, and refined sugar.

1½ cups blanched almond
   flour (page 29)

2 teaspoons baking powder

¼ teaspoon sea salt

2 large eggs,
   room temperature

¾ cup coconut sugar

¾ cup almond butter

1 teaspoon vanilla extract

1 cup paleo chocolate chips
   or chunks

1. Preheat the oven to 350°F. Line an 8-by-8-inch baking dish with parchment paper.

2. In a medium bowl, combine the almond flour, baking powder, and salt.

3. In a large bowl, beat the eggs, coconut sugar, almond butter, and vanilla until smooth and creamy.

4. Slowly pour the flour mixture into the wet ingredients and mix until evenly combined.

5. Fold in the chocolate chips, then pour the mixture into the prepared baking dish.

6. Bake for 20 minutes or until the top is golden brown. Cool completely before cutting and serving.

Prep Tip: Warm the eggs faster by immersing them in a bath of warm water.

PER SERVING (1 BROWNIE) CALORIES: 286; TOTAL FAT: 18G; SATURATED FAT: 3G; PROTEIN: 6G; TOTAL CARBOHYDRATES: 25G; FIBER: 5G; CHOLESTEROL: 31MG; MACROS: FAT: 57%; PROTEIN: 8%; CARBS: 35%

CHOCOLATE CHIP COCONUT BALLS

5 INGREDIENTS OR FEWER, EASY, EGG-FREE, QUICK PREP

MAKES 16 BALLS | PREP TIME: **10 MINUTES, PLUS 2 HOURS TO SET**

These homemade bite-size, no-bake coconut balls are full of nutrient-dense ingredients and are easy to make.

---

2 cups unsweetened shredded coconut

1 cup raw cashews

8 dates, pitted and chopped

½ cup paleo chocolate chips or chunks

½ cup coconut oil

1. Line a small edged baking sheet with parchment paper or wax paper.

2. In a food processor, pulse the shredded coconut, cashews, dates, chocolate chips, and coconut oil for 30 seconds or until evenly combined.

3. Roll the mixture into 1-inch balls and place onto the prepared baking sheet.

4. Set in the refrigerator for 2 hours or until hard. Serve.

> **Variation Tip:** Swap out chocolate chips for an equal amount of raisins or unsweetened dried cranberries.

PER SERVING (2 BALLS) CALORIES: 498; TOTAL FAT: 42G; SATURATED FAT: 30G; PROTEIN: 6G; TOTAL CARBOHYDRATES: 24G; FIBER: 7G; CHOLESTEROL: 0MG; MACROS: FAT: 76%; PROTEIN: 5%; CARBS: 19%

PECAN COOKIES

EASY, QUICK PREP, UNDER 30 MINUTES

MAKES 16 COOKIES | PREP TIME: 10 MINUTES | COOK TIME: 15 MINUTES

These pecan cookies smell just like the ones your grandma used to make, but they are free of grains and refined sugar.

1 cup blanched almond flour (page 29)

2 tablespoons coconut flour

½ teaspoon sea salt

½ cup coconut oil

½ cup coconut sugar

1 large egg, beaten

1 teaspoon vanilla extract

½ cup chopped raw pecans

1. Preheat the oven to 325°F. Line an edged baking sheet with parchment paper.

2. In a small bowl, combine the almond flour, coconut flour, and salt.

3. In a large bowl, beat the coconut oil and sugar until creamy and smooth, then add the egg and vanilla.

4. Add the dry ingredients to the wet ingredients. Mix well until evenly combined. Fold in the pecans.

5. Using a tablespoon, scoop the dough onto the prepared baking sheet and press slightly. Bake for 15 minutes or until browned.

6. Remove from the oven and cool before serving.

Variation Tip: Almond flour can be swapped out for an equal amount of pecan flour for a more intense pecan flavor.

PER SERVING (1 COOKIE) CALORIES: 152; TOTAL FAT: 12G; SATURATED FAT: 7G; PROTEIN: 2G; TOTAL CARBOHYDRATES: 9G; FIBER: 2G; CHOLESTEROL: 12MG; MACROS: FAT: 71%; PROTEIN: 5%; CARBS: 24%

MINT CHIP ICE CREAM

5 INGREDIENTS OR FEWER, AIP-FRIENDLY, ALLERGEN-FREE, EASY, EGG-FREE

MAKES 2 CUPS | PREP TIME: 20 MINUTES, PLUS 2 HOURS TO FREEZE

When I was growing up, one of my favorite ice cream flavors was mint chocolate chip. I wanted to create an ice cream similar to that, but one everyone could enjoy.

FOR THE CHOCOLATE

½ cup melted coconut oil

2 tablespoons pure maple syrup

1 tablespoon carob powder

FOR THE ICE CREAM

1 (13.5-ounce) can full-fat coconut milk

1 tablespoon pure maple syrup

½ teaspoon peppermint extract

TO MAKE THE CHOCOLATE

1. In a small bowl, whisk together the coconut oil, maple syrup, and carob. Put the bowl in the freezer for 20 minutes or until the chocolate has completely frozen.

2. Break the chocolate up into thin chunks with a fork.

TO MAKE THE ICE CREAM

1. Pour the coconut milk, syrup, and peppermint extract into a blender.

2. Blend on high for 30 seconds or until smooth with no more visible coconut fat.

3. Fold in the chocolate chunks and pour into a loaf pan.

4. Freeze the ice cream for 2 hours or until completely frozen. Serve immediately.

> **Storage Tip:** Store in an airtight freezer-safe container for up to 1 week in the freezer.

PER SERVING (½ CUP) CALORIES: 527; TOTAL FAT: 50G; SATURATED FAT: 44G; PROTEIN: 2G; TOTAL CARBOHYDRATES: 18G; FIBER: 3G; CHOLESTEROL: 0MG; MACROS: FAT: 85%; PROTEIN: 2%; CARBS: 13%

PUMPKIN PIE BITES

EASY, QUICK PREP

MAKES 32 BITES | PREP TIME: **10 MINUTES** | COOK TIME: **25 MINUTES**

Packed full of pumpkin pie flavor but free of refined sugar, these bites make for a perfect fall treat.

FOR THE COATING

¼ cup coconut sugar

3 teaspoons ground pumpkin pie spice

FOR THE PUMPKIN PIE BITES

Coconut oil cooking spray

2 cups blanched almond flour (page 29)

2 teaspoons baking powder

1 teaspoon ground pumpkin pie spice

½ teaspoon ground nutmeg

½ teaspoon sea salt

1 cup pumpkin purée

½ cup coconut sugar

1 large egg

½ cup full-fat coconut milk

¼ cup melted coconut oil

1 teaspoon vanilla extract

TO MAKE THE COATING

In a small bowl, whisk together the coconut sugar and pumpkin pie spice. Set aside.

TO MAKE THE PUMPKIN PIE BITES

1. Preheat the oven to 350°F. Lightly grease the cups in a mini-muffin tin with cooking spray.

2. In a large bowl, combine the almond flour, baking powder, pumpkin pie spice, nutmeg, and salt.

3. In another large bowl, whisk together the pumpkin purée, coconut sugar, egg, coconut milk, coconut oil, and vanilla.

4. Slowly mix the dry ingredients into the wet ingredients, stirring to combine.

5. Using a tablespoon, spoon the mixture into each muffin cup.

6. Bake for 20 to 25 minutes or until puffed and golden.

7. Allow to cool completely before removing from the pan.

8. Roll each pumpkin pie bite in the coating and serve immediately.

> **Ingredient Tip:** Make a homemade pumpkin pie spice by combining 4 teaspoons of ground cinnamon, 2 teaspoons of ground ginger, 1 teaspoon of ground cloves, and ½ teaspoon of ground nutmeg.

PER SERVING (2 BITES) CALORIES: 145; TOTAL FAT: 9G; SATURATED FAT: 5G; PROTEIN: 3G; TOTAL CARBOHYDRATES: 13G; FIBER: 2G; CHOLESTEROL: 12MG; MACROS: FAT: 56%; PROTEIN: 8%; CARBS: 36%

PECAN PIE BARS

EASY, EGG-FREE, QUICK PREP

MAKES 12 BARS | PREP TIME: 10 MINUTES, PLUS 2 HOURS TO SET | COOK TIME: 35 MINUTES

Enjoy this dessert's shortbread-like crust and caramelized pecan filling. These bars will leave your taste buds dancing for more.

FOR THE CRUST

**2 cups blanched almond
flour (page 29)**

⅓ cup melted coconut oil

¼ cup pure maple syrup

1 teaspoon vanilla extract

¼ teaspoon sea salt

FOR THE FILLING

½ cup coconut sugar

¼ cup pure maple syrup

¼ cup coconut oil

1 teaspoon vanilla extract

1 tablespoon almond milk

2½ cups chopped pecans

TO MAKE THE CRUST

1. Preheat the oven to 350°F. Line an 8-by-8-inch baking dish with parchment paper.

2. In a medium bowl, combine the almond flour, coconut oil, maple syrup, vanilla, and salt.

3. Press the mixture into the bottom of the prepared baking dish and bake for 15 minutes or until the top is light golden brown. Allow the crust to cool completely before filling. Leave the oven on.

TO MAKE THE FILLING

1. While the crust is baking, in a medium saucepan, whisk together the coconut sugar, maple syrup, coconut oil, and vanilla over medium heat for 5 minutes or until it reaches a gentle boil.

2. Turn the burner off and fold in the almond milk and pecans.

3. Pour the filling in the crust and bake for 20 minutes or until the filling has solidified and is no longer runny.

4. Allow the pecan pie bars to cool before setting in the refrigerator for 2 hours. Cut and serve.

> **Variation Tip:** Almond milk can be swapped out for an equal amount of coconut milk.

PER SERVING (1 BAR) CALORIES: 391; TOTAL FAT: 31G; SATURATED FAT: 12G; PROTEIN: 5G; TOTAL CARBOHYDRATES: 23G; FIBER: 4G; CHOLESTEROL: 0MG; MACROS: FAT: 71%; PROTEIN: 5%; CARBS: 24%

CHOCOLATE, ALMOND, AND SEA SALT FUDGE

5 INGREDIENTS OR FEWER, EASY, EGG-FREE, QUICK PREP

MAKES 16 PIECES | PREP TIME: **5 MINUTES, PLUS 2 HOURS TO SET** | COOK TIME: **5 MINUTES**

Ditch the store-bought fudge and opt for a treat free of refined sugar and dairy.

½ cup coconut oil

½ cup almond butter

½ cup cacao powder

¼ cup pure maple syrup

½ teaspoon coarse sea salt

1. Line a loaf pan with parchment paper or wax paper.

2. In a small saucepan, whisk together the coconut oil, almond butter, cacao powder, and maple syrup over medium heat for 5 minutes or until the coconut oil is completely melted.

3. Pour into the prepared pan and sprinkle with salt. Set in the freezer for 2 hours or until hardened.

4. Remove the parchment paper from the pan and cut into 16 pieces before serving.

> Variation Tip: For an allergen-free dessert, swap out the almond butter for sunflower butter.

PER SERVING (1 PIECE) CALORIES: 169; TOTAL FAT: 13G; SATURATED FAT: 8G; PROTEIN: 3G; TOTAL CARBOHYDRATES: 10G; FIBER: 3G; CHOLESTEROL: 0MG; MACROS: FAT: 69%; PROTEIN: 7%; CARBS: 24%

CHOCOLATE MUFFINS

MAKES 6 LARGE MUFFINS | PREP TIME: **10 MINUTES** | COOK TIME: **30 MINUTES**

Your family will think you picked these chocolate muffins up from the bakery—they're *that* indulgent!

Coconut oil cooking spray

1 cup blanched almond
    flour (page 29)

½ cup coconut sugar

¼ cup cacao powder

1 tablespoon coconut flour

1 tablespoon arrowroot flour

2 teaspoons baking soda

¼ teaspoon sea salt

½ cup warm water

2 large eggs,
    room temperature

3 tablespoons avocado oil

2 teaspoons vanilla extract

1. Preheat the oven to 350°F. Line a muffin tin with liners and lightly grease the liners with cooking spray.

2. In a large bowl, combine the almond flour, coconut sugar, cacao powder, coconut flour, arrowroot flour, baking soda, and salt.

3. In a medium bowl, whisk together the water, eggs, avocado oil, and vanilla.

4. Combine the dry ingredients with the wet ingredients.

5. Using a ⅓-cup measuring cup, scoop the batter into the muffin cups.

6. Bake for 30 minutes or until the tops have risen and are firm to the touch. Remove from the oven. Cool completely before serving.

> Prep Tip: Warm eggs faster by immersing them in a bath of warm water.

PER SERVING (1 MUFFIN) CALORIES: 293; TOTAL FAT: 17G; SATURATED FAT: 4G; PROTEIN: 8G; TOTAL CARBOHYDRATES: 27G; FIBER: 6G; CHOLESTEROL: 62MG; MACROS: FAT: 52%; PROTEIN: 11%; CARBS: 37%

CHOCOLATE-AVOCADO PUDDING

AIP-FRIENDLY, ALLERGEN-FREE, EASY, EGG-FREE, NUT-FREE, QUICK PREP

SERVES 2 | PREP TIME: **5 MINUTES, PLUS 1 HOUR TO CHILL**

Curb your sweet tooth with this velvety smooth and decadent chocolate-avocado pudding.

1 medium ripe avocado, peeled and pitted

¼ cup cacao powder

2 tablespoons pure maple syrup

¼ teaspoon vanilla extract

1. Put the avocado, cacao powder, maple syrup, and vanilla into a blender.

2. Blend on high for 1 minute or until no avocado clumps remain. Pour into a medium bowl.

3. Chill the pudding for 1 hour in the refrigerator before serving.

> Variation Tip: The maple syrup can be swapped out for an equal amount of raw honey.

PER SERVING CALORIES: 190; TOTAL FAT: 12G; SATURATED FAT: 2G; PROTEIN: 3G; TOTAL CARBOHYDRATES: 25G; FIBER: 8G; CHOLESTEROL: 0MG; MACROS: FAT: 53%; PROTEIN: 4%; CARBS: 43%

LEMON BARS

EASY, QUICK PREP

MAKES 12 BARS | PREP TIME: **10 MINUTES, PLUS 2 HOURS TO SET** | COOK TIME: **30 MINUTES**
Enjoy your favorite lemony dessert by using this easy-to-make, richly tart recipe.

FOR THE CRUST

Coconut oil cooking spray

2 cups blanched almond flour (page 29)

⅓ cup melted coconut oil

¼ cup raw honey

1 teaspoon vanilla extract

¼ teaspoon sea salt

FOR THE FILLING

½ cup raw honey

½ cup freshly squeezed lemon juice (about 2 large lemons)

3 large eggs

1 large egg yolk

Zest of 1 lemon

1 tablespoon arrowroot flour

1 teaspoon coconut flour

TO MAKE THE CRUST

1. Preheat the oven to 350°F. Lightly grease an 8-by-8-inch baking dish with cooking spray.

2. In a medium bowl, combine the almond flour, coconut oil, honey, vanilla, and salt.

3. Press the mixture into the bottom of the prepared baking dish and bake for 15 minutes or until the top is a light golden brown. (Leave the oven on.) Allow the crust to cool completely before filling.

TO MAKE THE FILLING

1. While the crust is baking, in a medium bowl, whisk together the honey, lemon juice, eggs and yolk, lemon zest, arrowroot flour, and coconut flour until smooth and creamy.

2. Pour the filling into the crust and bake for 15 minutes or until the center has set and is no longer runny.

3. Remove from the oven and let cool before setting in the refrigerator for 2 hours. Cut and serve.

Storage Tip: Store in the refrigerator in an airtight container for up to 3 days.

PER SERVING (1 BAR) CALORIES: 217; TOTAL FAT: 13G; SATURATED FAT: 6G; PROTEIN: 4G; TOTAL CARBOHYDRATES: 21G; FIBER: 1G; CHOLESTEROL: 64MG; MACROS: FAT: 54%; PROTEIN: 7%; CARBS: 39%

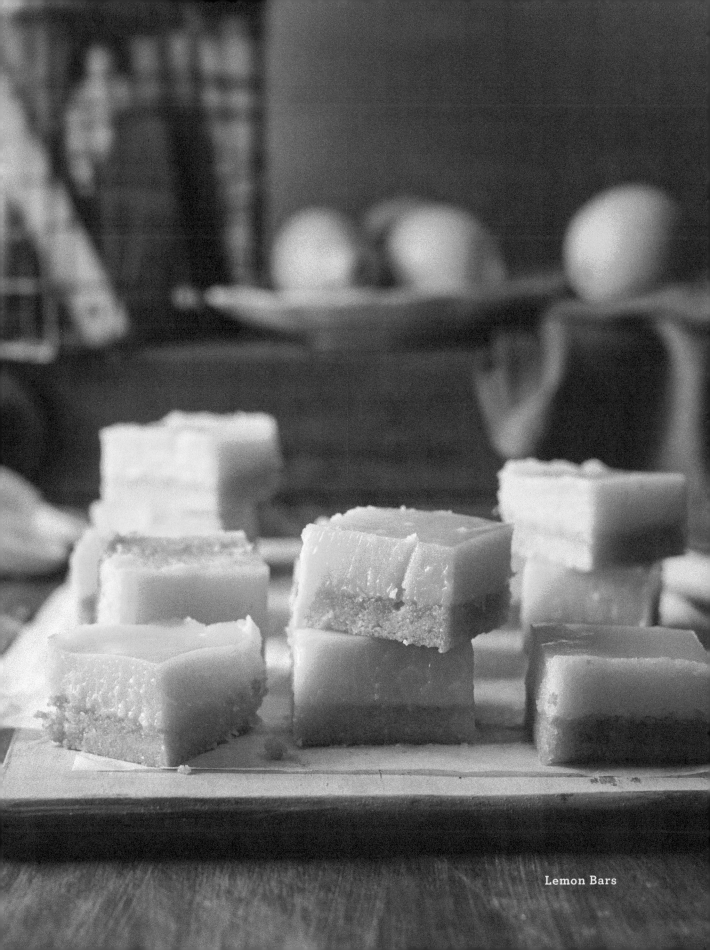

Lemon Bars

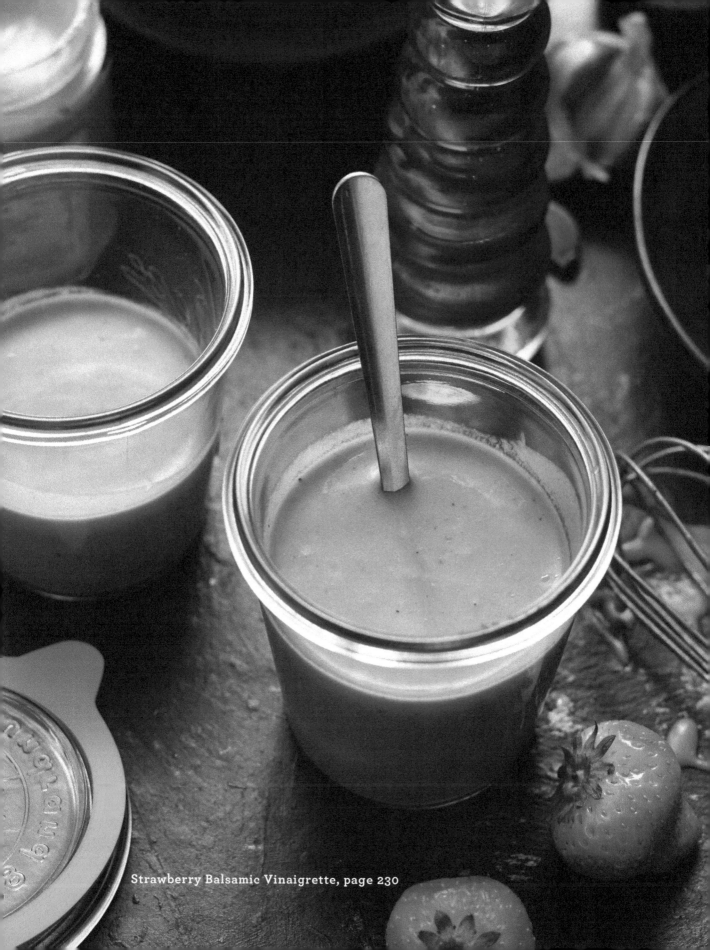

Strawberry Balsamic Vinaigrette, page 230

CHAPTER FOURTEEN

DRESSINGS, SAUCES, AND SEASONINGS

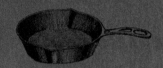

STRAWBERRY BALSAMIC VINAIGRETTE

MAKES 1 CUP | PREP TIME: 5 MINUTES

This dressing can be used as a marinade for chicken or drizzled over Strawberry-Walnut Summer Salad (page 90).

1 cup chopped
  fresh strawberries

¼ cup extra-virgin olive oil
  or avocado oil

¼ cup balsamic vinegar

1 tablespoon Dijon mustard

1 medium garlic
  clove, minced

¼ teaspoon sea salt

¼ teaspoon freshly ground
  black pepper

1. Put the strawberries, olive oil, balsamic vinegar, mustard, garlic, salt, and pepper into a blender.

2. Blend on high for 1 minute or until smooth with no visible strawberry chunks. Serve immediately.

> **Storage Tip:** Store in an airtight container in the refrigerator for up to 2 days.

PER SERVING (2 TABLESPOONS) CALORIES: 62; TOTAL FAT: 6G; SATURATED FAT: 1G; PROTEIN: 0G; TOTAL CARBOHYDRATES: 2G; FIBER: 1G; CHOLESTEROL: 0MG; MACROS: FAT: 87%; PROTEIN: 2%; CARBS: 11%

TWO-MINUTE TACO SEASONING

ALLERGEN-FREE, EASY, EGG-FREE, NUT-FREE, QUICK PREP, UNDER 30 MINUTES

MAKES ¼ CUP | PREP TIME: **5 MINUTES**

Make every night taco night with this no-mess, filler-free taco seasoning.

1 tablespoon chili powder

1 tablespoon ground cumin

1 teaspoon freshly ground
   black pepper

1 teaspoon ground paprika

1 teaspoon garlic powder

1 teaspoon onion powder

½ teaspoon dried oregano

½ teaspoon sea salt

¼ teaspoon red pepper
   flakes (optional)

In a small bowl, combine the chili powder, cumin, pepper, paprika, garlic powder, onion powder, oregano, salt, and red pepper flakes (if using).

Storage Tip: Store in an airtight container in a cool and dark cabinet for up to 6 months. Double or triple the recipe to have more on hand as needed.

PER SERVING (1½ TEASPOONS) CALORIES: 10; TOTAL FAT: 0G; SATURATED FAT: 0G; PROTEIN: 0G; TOTAL CARBOHYDRATES: 2G; FIBER: 1G; CHOLESTEROL: 0MG; MACROS FAT: 10%; PROTEIN: 10%; CARBS: 80%

ZESTY ITALIAN SEASONING

AIP-FRIENDLY, ALLERGEN-FREE, EASY, EGG-FREE, NUT-FREE, QUICK PREP,
UNDER 30 MINUTES

MAKES ½ CUP | PREP TIME: 5 MINUTES

As the basis for many Italian-inspired dishes, this is a useful and versatile seasoning mix to have on hand.

1½ tablespoons dried basil

1½ tablespoons
   dried oregano

1 tablespoon dried thyme

1 tablespoon dried rosemary

1½ teaspoons
   ground marjoram

1 teaspoon garlic powder

¾ teaspoon dried sage

In a small bowl, combine the basil, oregano, thyme, rosemary, marjoram, garlic powder, and sage.

> **Make-Ahead Tip:** Double the recipe and store extra seasoning in an airtight container in a cool, dark cabinet for up to 6 months.

PER SERVING (1½ TEASPOONS) CALORIES: 3; TOTAL FAT: 0G; SATURATED FAT: 0G; PROTEIN: 0G; TOTAL CARBOHYDRATES: 1G; FIBER: 0G; CHOLESTEROL: 0MG; MACROS: FAT: 2%; PROTEIN: 2%; CARBS: 96%

EVERYTHING BAGEL SEASONING

MAKES ½ CUP | PREP TIME: 5 MINUTES

Ditch the notion that this seasoning is strictly for bagels and top your favorite protein with this seedy blend.

2 tablespoons poppy seeds

2 tablespoons white
   sesame seeds

1 tablespoon dried
   minced garlic

1 tablespoon dried
   minced onion

2 teaspoons coarse sea salt

In a small bowl, combine the poppy seeds, sesame seeds, garlic, onion, and salt.

> **Storage Tip:** Store in an airtight container in a cool, dark cabinet for up to 3 months.

PER SERVING (1½ TEASPOONS) CALORIES: 16; TOTAL FAT: 1G; SATURATED FAT: 0G; PROTEIN: 1G; TOTAL CARBOHYDRATES: 1G; FIBER: 0G; CHOLESTEROL: 0MG; MACROS: FAT: 60%; PROTEIN: 15%; CARBS: 25%

REAL PALEO MAYONNAISE

MAKES 1 CUP | PREP TIME: 10 MINUTES

The key to making this mayo perfect is using extra-light olive oil or avocado oil and slowly drizzling it in to produce smooth results.

---

1 large egg,
  room temperature

1 cup extra-light olive oil or
  avocado oil, divided

1 teaspoon ground mustard

½ teaspoon sea salt

1 tablespoon freshly
  squeezed lemon juice

1. In a food processor, blend the egg, ¼ cup of olive oil, the mustard, and salt on high for 30 seconds or until pale yellow.

2. Slowly drizzle in the remaining ¾ cup of olive oil until the mayonnaise becomes emulsified and thick.

3. Fold in the lemon juice. Serve immediately.

> **Storage Tip:** Store in an airtight container in the refrigerator for up to 1 week.

PER SERVING (1 TABLESPOON) CALORIES: 114; TOTAL FAT: 12G; SATURATED FAT: 2G; PROTEIN: 1G; TOTAL CARBOHYDRATES: 0G; FIBER: 0G; CHOLESTEROL: 12MG; MACROS: FAT: 95%; PROTEIN: 4%; CARBS: 1%

SUGAR-FREE KETCHUP

ALLERGEN-FREE, EASY, EGG-FREE, QUICK PREP, UNDER 30 MINUTES

MAKES 1 CUP | PREP TIME: **5 MINUTES** | COOK TIME: **5 MINUTES**

This easy-to-make homemade ketchup uses staples from your paleo pantry and requires minimal prep work.

---

1 (6-ounce) can
   tomato paste

¼ cup tomato sauce

2 tablespoons
   coconut aminos

1 tablespoon apple
   cider vinegar

½ teaspoon garlic powder

½ teaspoon onion powder

¼ teaspoon sea salt

1. In a small saucepan, combine the tomato paste and tomato sauce over medium heat for 3 minutes or until fragrant and warm.

2. Whisk in the coconut aminos, apple cider vinegar, garlic powder, onion powder, and salt for 1 minute or until the ketchup is thick and smooth.

3. Remove the ketchup from the burner and cool before serving or storing.

> **Storage Tip:** Store in an airtight container in the refrigerator for up to 2 weeks.

PER SERVING (2 TABLESPOONS) CALORIES: 25; TOTAL FAT: 0G; SATURATED FAT: 0G; PROTEIN: 1G; TOTAL CARBOHYDRATES: 6G; FIBER: 1G; CHOLESTEROL: 0MG; MACROS: FAT: 1%; PROTEIN: 11%; CARBS: 88%

CREAMY RANCH DRESSING

EASY, QUICK PREP, UNDER 30 MINUTES

MAKES 1 CUP | PREP TIME: 5 MINUTES, PLUS 1 HOUR TO CHILL

This dressing is perfect for dipping your favorite vegetables, marinating chicken, or pouring over my favorite, Grilled Buffalo Chicken Salad (page 93).

½ cup Real Paleo
  Mayonnaise (page 234)

¼ cup full-fat coconut milk

1 teaspoon dried parsley

½ teaspoon garlic powder

½ teaspoon onion powder

½ teaspoon dried dill

½ teaspoon dried chives

¼ teaspoon sea salt

¼ teaspoon freshly ground
  black pepper

1. In a small bowl, whisk together the mayonnaise, coconut milk, parsley, garlic powder, onion powder, dill, chives, salt, and pepper for 1 minute or until smooth and creamy.

2. Transfer to an airtight container and refrigerate for 1 hour before serving.

Storage Tip: Store in an airtight container in the refrigerator for up to 1 week.

PER SERVING (2 TABLESPOONS) CALORIES: 134; TOTAL FAT: 14G; SATURATED FAT: 4G; PROTEIN: 1G; TOTAL CARBOHYDRATES: 1G; FIBER: 0G; CHOLESTEROL: 12MG; MACROS: FAT: 94%; PROTEIN: 3%; CARBS: 3%

DATE-INFUSED BARBECUE SAUCE

ALLERGEN-FREE, EASY, EGG-FREE, QUICK PREP, UNDER 30 MINUTES

MAKES 2 CUPS | PREP TIME: 10 MINUTES | COOK TIME: 5 MINUTES

You'll want to smother all your meats (and even some veggies!) in this delicious and easy-to-make barbecue sauce.

8 Medjool dates, pitted

1 (6-ounce) can tomato paste

½ cup water

¼ cup balsamic vinegar

2 tablespoons coconut aminos

2 tablespoons Dijon mustard

½ teaspoon onion powder

½ teaspoon garlic powder

½ teaspoon sea salt

½ teaspoon freshly ground black pepper

1. In a medium saucepan, whisk together the dates, tomato paste, water, balsamic vinegar, coconut aminos, mustard, onion powder, garlic powder, salt, and pepper over medium-high heat for 5 minutes or until the dates are soft.

2. Blend the mixture in a food processor on high speed for 1 to 2 minutes or until the sauce becomes smooth and thick. Serve immediately.

Storage Tip: Store in an airtight container in the refrigerator for up to 2 weeks.

PER SERVING (2 TABLESPOONS) CALORIES: 60; TOTAL FAT: 0G; SATURATED FAT: 0G; PROTEIN: 1G; TOTAL CARBOHYDRATES: 14G; FIBER: 2G; CHOLESTEROL: 0MG; MACROS: FAT: 0%; PROTEIN: 7%; CARBS: 93%

MAPLE BALSAMIC VINAIGRETTE

5 INGREDIENTS OR FEWER, AIP-FRIENDLY, ALLERGEN-FREE, EASY, EGG-FREE, NUT-FREE, QUICK PREP, UNDER 30 MINUTES

MAKES 1 CUP | PREP TIME: 5 MINUTES

This dressing is perfect for marinating chicken or adding to any autumnal salad.

¾ cup extra-light olive oil or avocado oil

¼ cup balsamic vinegar

3 tablespoons pure maple syrup

1 tablespoon Dijon mustard

⅛ teaspoon sea salt

In a small bowl, whisk together the olive oil, balsamic vinegar, maple syrup, mustard, and salt for 1 minute or until the oil and vinegar are no longer separated. Serve immediately.

Storage Tip: Store in an airtight container in the refrigerator for up to 2 weeks.

PER SERVING (2 TABLESPOONS) CALORIES: 199; TOTAL FAT: 19G; SATURATED FAT: 3G; PROTEIN: 0G; TOTAL CARBOHYDRATES: 7G; FIBER: 0G; CHOLESTEROL: 0MG; MACROS: FAT: 86%; PROTEIN: 1%; CARBS: 13%

MUSHROOM GRAVY

AIP-FRIENDLY, ALLERGEN-FREE, EASY, EGG-FREE, NUT-FREE, QUICK PREP,
UNDER 30 MINUTES

MAKES 2 CUPS | PREP TIME: **10 MINUTES** | COOK TIME: **15 MINUTES**

Enjoy the earthiness of the mushrooms mixed with savory beef broth and seasoned by subtle hints of fresh rosemary.

1 tablespoon avocado oil

2 cups chopped
  cremini mushrooms

1 small white onion, diced

2 medium garlic
  cloves, minced

2 cups Beef Bone Broth
  (page 27)

1 tablespoon finely chopped
  fresh rosemary

¼ teaspoon sea salt

¼ teaspoon freshly ground
  black pepper

3 tablespoons
  arrowroot flour

3 tablespoons warm water

1. In a medium skillet, heat the avocado oil over medium heat for 5 minutes or until the oil starts to shimmer.

2. Sauté the mushrooms, onion, and garlic for 5 minutes or until lightly browned.

3. Add the bone broth, rosemary, salt, and pepper.

4. Deglaze the skillet, stirring to scrape up the browned bits from the bottom, while bringing the gravy to a gentle boil. Turn the burner off.

5. In a small bowl, whisk together the arrowroot flour and water for 20 seconds or until smooth. Pour the mixture into the gravy and whisk for 1 minute or until the gravy starts to thicken. Let stand for 5 minutes before serving.

> **Variation Tip:** For a creamy gravy, put the finished mushroom gravy into a food processor and blend for 1 minute or until smooth.

PER SERVING (3 TABLESPOONS) CALORIES: 38; TOTAL FAT: 2G; SATURATED FAT: 0G; PROTEIN: 2G; TOTAL CARBOHYDRATES: 3G; FIBER: 1G; CHOLESTEROL: 2MG; MACROS: FAT: 47%; PROTEIN: 22%; CARBS: 31%

GARDEN-FRESH SPAGHETTI SAUCE

ALLERGEN-FREE, EASY, EGG-FREE, NUT-FREE

MAKES 4 CUPS | PREP TIME: **15 MINUTES** | COOK TIME: **1 HOUR**

Enjoy the traditional basil flavor of Grandma's sauce with sweet cherry tomatoes in every bite!

3 pounds cherry tomatoes

4 tablespoons avocado oil, divided

1 small white onion, diced

5 medium garlic cloves, minced

5 fresh basil leaves

3 thyme sprigs

1 teaspoon sea salt

1 teaspoon freshly ground black pepper

1. Preheat the oven to 400°F. Line a 12-by-17-inch edged baking sheet with parchment paper.

2. In a large bowl, combine the tomatoes and 1 tablespoon of avocado oil. Arrange the tomatoes onto the baking sheet and bake for 30 minutes or until most of the tomatoes have split.

3. In the meantime, heat the remaining 3 tablespoons of avocado oil in a large stockpot over medium heat for 3 minutes or until the oil starts to shimmer.

4. Sauté the onion and garlic for 2 minutes or until the onion is translucent.

5. Add the cooked tomatoes with their juices, basil, thyme, salt, and pepper.

6. Cover, reduce the heat to low, and simmer for 25 minutes or until the tomatoes look mushy. Remove from the heat and let cool.

7. Transfer the sauce to a food processor and blend on high for 1 minute or until the sauce is smooth. (Depending on the food processor's capacity, the sauce may need to be blended in batches.) Serve immediately.

> **Storage Tip:** Store the spaghetti sauce in an airtight container in the refrigerator for up to 1 week or freeze in a freezer-safe container for up to 6 months.

PER SERVING (½ CUP) CALORIES: 103; TOTAL FAT: 7G; SATURATED FAT: 1G; PROTEIN: 2G; TOTAL CARBOHYDRATES: 8G; FIBER: 2G; CHOLESTEROL: 0MG; MACROS: FAT: 61%; PROTEIN: 8%; CARBS: 31%

CHIMICHURRI SAUCE

ALLERGEN-FREE, EASY, EGG-FREE, NUT-FREE, QUICK PREP, UNDER 30 MINUTES

MAKES 1 CUP | PREP TIME: 5 MINUTES

This sauce makes the perfect marinade or topping for Chimichurri Pan-Seared Rib Eye (page 174) or Chimichurri Baked Chicken Breast (page 131).

1 cup fresh cilantro leaves

¼ cup avocado oil

¼ cup red wine vinegar

3 small garlic cloves, peeled

½ teaspoon red pepper flakes

¼ teaspoon sea salt

¼ teaspoon freshly ground black pepper

In a food processor, pulse the cilantro, avocado oil, red wine vinegar, garlic, red pepper flakes, salt, and pepper for 30 to 45 seconds or until smooth but still slightly chunky. Serve immediately.

> **Storage Tip:** Store the chimichurri sauce in an airtight container in the refrigerator for up to 2 days or freeze in small amounts in ice cube trays for up to 3 months and defrost as needed.

PER SERVING (2 TABLESPOONS) CALORIES: 67; TOTAL FAT: 7G; SATURATED FAT: 1G; PROTEIN: 0G; TOTAL CARBOHYDRATES: 1G; FIBER: 0G; CHOLESTEROL: 0MG; MACROS: FAT: 94%; PROTEIN: 0%; CARBS: 6%

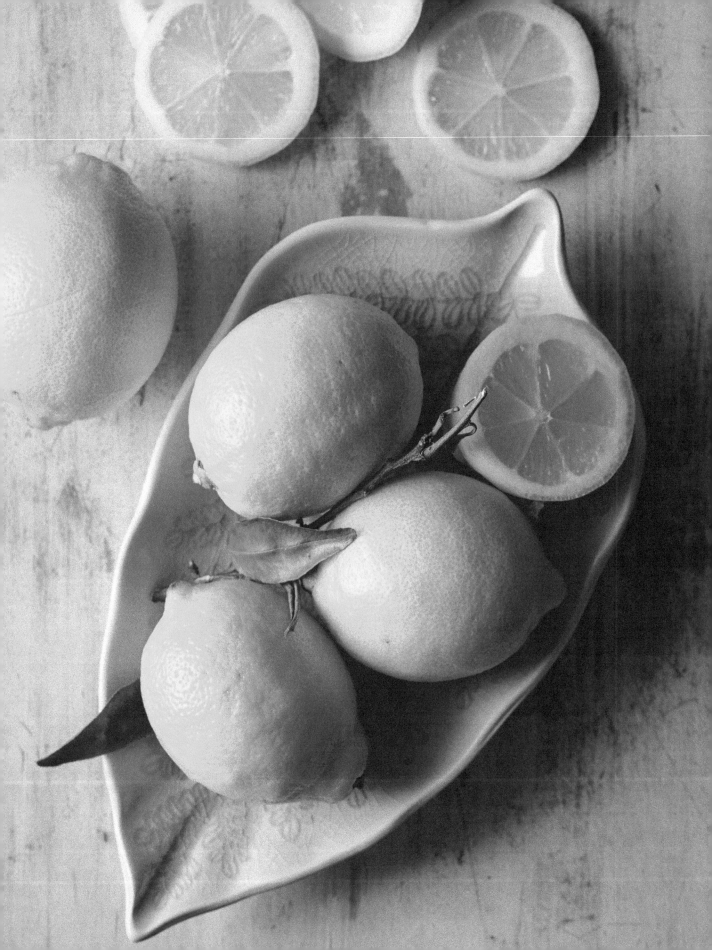

RESOURCES

WEBSITES

Amazon: Paleo foods and essentials
    www.amazon.com/shop/momeatspaleo
Calorie Calculator
    www.calculator.net/calorie-calculator.html
Macronutrient Calculator
    www.calculator.net/macro-calculator.html
Mark's Daily Apple: Primal living and keto lifestyle blog
    www.marksdailyapple.com
Midwest Primal Health and Wellness: Health coaching
    www.midwestprimalhealthandwellness.com
Mom Eats Paleo: Recipes and lifestyle blog
    www.momeatspaleo.com
Paleo Leap: Information and recipes
    www.paleoleap.com
The Paleo Mom: Recipes and lifestyle blog
    www.thepaleomom.com
Primal Kitchen: Paleo foods and recipes
    www.primalkitchen.com
Serenity Kids: Paleo baby food
    www.myserenitykids.com
Thrive Market: Paleo foods
    www.thrivemarket.com/diets/paleo-diet
Wellness Mama: Natural health and lifestyle resources
    www.wellnessmama.com

BOOKS

Eat the Yolks by Liz Wolfe

Grain Brain: The Surprising Truth about Wheat, Carbs, and Sugar—Your Brain's Silent Killers by Dr. David Perlmutter

Paleo Family Meals and Kitchen Tips by Angela Blanchard

Paleo Kid's Edition Cookbook by Angela Blanchard

The Paleo Solution: The Original Human Diet by Robb Wolf

Practical Paleo: A Customized Approach to Health and a Whole-Foods Lifestyle by Diane Sanfilippo

The Primal Blueprint by Mark Sisson

Transitioning and Maintaining the Paleo Lifestyle: Healthy for Life by Angela Blanchard

Weight Loss on Paleo: Going Beyond the Scale by Angela Blanchard

SUGGESTED PALEO-APPROVED BRANDS

Applegate
Artisana Organics
Birch Benders
Cappello's
Coconut Secret
Dry Farm Wines
Epic
FitVine
Great Lakes
Julian Bakery
Justin's
Kettle & Fire
Lärabar

Mavuno Harvest
Mission Meats
Muir Glen
Native Forest
Paleonola
Primal Kitchen
Primal Palate
Serenity Kids
Siete
Simple Mills
SunButter
Tessemae's

REFERENCES

Calder, Philip C., and Robert F. Grimble. "Polyunsaturated Fatty Acids, Inflammation and Immunity." *European Journal of Clinical Nutrition* 56 (2002): S14–S19. https://doi.org/10.1038/sj.ejcn.1601478.

Norwood, R., Tegan Cruwys, Veronique S. Chachay, and J. Sheffield. "The Psychological Characteristics of People Consuming Vegetarian, Vegan, Paleo, Gluten Free and Weight Loss Dietary Patterns." *Obesity Science and Practice* 5, no. 2 (February 2019): 148–58. https://doi.org/10.1002/osp4.325.

Paleo Leap (blog). "Keto and Paleo Macros: 5 Different Macronutrient Ratio Options to Consider." Accessed October 28, 2019. https://paleoleap.com/keto-paleo-5-macronutrient-ratio-options.

Soliman, Ghada A. "Dietary Cholesterol and the Lack of Evidence in Cardiovascular Disease." *Nutrients* 10, no. 6 (June 2018): 780. https://doi.org/10.3390/nu10060780.

University Health News. "Three Benefits Paleo Diet Followers Enjoy in Just 10 Days." Accessed October 28, 2019. https://universityhealthnews.com/daily/heart-health/paleo-diet-benefits-include-improved-cholesterol-triglycerides-blood-pressure-and-insulin-levels-after-only-10-days.

Volk, Brittanie M., Laura J. Kunces, Daniel J. Freidenreich, Brian R. Kupchak, Catherine Saenz, Juan C. Artistizabal, Maria Luz Fernanadez, et al. "Effects of Step-Wise Increases in Dietary Carbohydrate on Circulating Saturated Fatty Acids and Palmitoleic Acid in Adults with Metabolic Syndrome." *PLOS ONE* 9, no. 11 (November 2014): e113605. https://doi.org/10.1371/journal.pone.0113605.

Zioudrou, Christine, Richard A. Streaty, and Werner A. Klee. "Opioid Peptides Derived from Food Proteins: The Exorphins." *Journal of Biological Chemistry* 254, no. 7 (April 1979): 2446–49. https://www.ncbi.nlm.nih.gov/pubmed/372181.

RECIPE INDEX

INDEX

ACKNOWLEDGMENTS

I want to take a moment to thank all those who helped me get to where I am today in life and helped make this book happen. I'll probably forget someone, but don't take it personally—your help and support are much appreciated. Here it goes, in no particular order.

First, I have to thank Callisto Media for giving me the opportunity to write this book and for their trust in me to provide my expertise and knowledge of the paleo diet and lifestyle. Also, thanks to everyone involved who helped make this book happen at Callisto Media. You rock!

Secondly, if it wasn't for my husband and his continued support throughout my journey and the making of this book, I honestly don't think I would be where I am today. His unconditional love and drive for my success is my motivation in life. I love you!

Thirdly, I'd like to thank my mom and dad for bringing me into this world. If it weren't for them, there would be no me, which would be a great disappointment to many. I also have to thank them for putting up with my shenanigans growing up and for their unconditional love.

Next, I have to give my kids some credit in all this. They are the reason for my complete lifestyle change and my passion for helping others achieve optimal health and wellness through the paleo diet and lifestyle.

I'd also like to thank all my followers and readers at Mom Eats Paleo—your likes, shares, and comments bring a smile to my face. Please continue, and know you don't go unnoticed!

Lastly, I'd like to give a shout out to the rest of my family and friends who have been there from the beginning. Thank you!

ABOUT THE AUTHOR

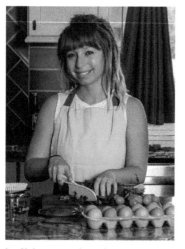

Angela Blanchard is a Certified Primal Health Coach and Personal Trainer, a professional blogger at Mom Eats Paleo, and business owner of Midwest Primal Health and Wellness. In addition to *The Big Book of Paleo Cooking*, Angela has many self-publications, including *Weight Loss on Paleo* and her *Kid's Edition Cookbook*, which can be found on her website along with other titles. Angela resides in Wisconsin with her husband, two boys, and two English bulldogs. In her free time, she enjoys long periods of silence, an occasional adult beverage, and binge-watching crime documentaries, but you'll usually find her in the kitchen cooking up something new and exciting.

CPSIA information can be obtained
at www.ICGtesting.com
Printed in the USA
LVHW012357160220
646996LV00001B/1